MW01675356

THE ESSENTIAL AIR FRYER COOKBOOK FOR BEGINNERS:

600 Easy and Delicious Air Fryer Recipes | With Vegan and Vegetarian Recipes

ISBN: 9798634999524

Warning-Disclaimer

The purpose of this book is to educate and entertain. The author or publisher does not guarantee that anyone following the techniques, suggestions, tips, ideas, or strategies will become successful. The author and publisher shall have neither liability or responsibility to anyone with respect to any loss or damage cause, or alleged to be cause, directly or indirectly by the information contained in this book.

TABLE OF CONTENTS

INTRODUCTION

Cooking simple, safe and delightful home-made meals has become more feasible with a groundbreaking kitchen gadget such as the air fryer. It will not only focus on saving time but also more importantly, in your diet, you will drastically cut on oil.

What's an air fryer?

Till we continue, you can know what actually an air fryer is. The air fryer has begun production in 2010, which is essentially a kitchen gadget that is cooking without oil. As little oil as necessary, as need be. Perhaps by rapidly spreading hot air with an integrated fan, a method which generates temperatures that are high sufficiently replicate traditional frying.

After this, air fryers can microwave food without including the risks of conventional oil frying–other than oil burning or massive damage–and could do it very consistently, even controlled.

Practical concepts

Because an air fryer uses hot air, others might argue that it functions the same way as a traditional oven. One should always note, though, that both devices lead to a different performance, mostly because of their technical variations.

Whereas the ovens explicitly add the dry air and heat to the food but require a little more time for cooking, air fryers use a mechanism that easily ripples air across the plate, allowing in quick cooking times but have a crispier look.

When and how to use an Air Fryer

An air fryer uses hot air, some may even say that it actually works very much the same as traditional ovens. Nonetheless, one must also note that the same devices yield different outcomes, mostly because of their technical variations.

- Using the appropriate extension. Clear up any confusion with the recipe, before everything, which adapter you would need for the recipe. Need a blender? A Barbecue? And some extra pan? Make sure you've got everything packed.
- Unpasted your cup. Although air fryers may not require oil to operate, not to use oil also represents a higher risk that some dishes may stick to the container or bowl. That being said, for a genuine oil-free option, you could either spray the tray lightly with oil to prevent your food from stuck or add baking paper to the above. All the same, it's essential to untick your cup.
- Level configuration. If you want to use Fahrenheit, Celsius or quantity of voltage, make sure to place the frying pan at the right consistency or voltage intensity so it won't over or sear steaks your platter. Many air fryers often have "modes" for other types of foods like chips and cakes, or cooking variants.
- Bringing the timer on. When the temperature is over, simply set a timer as stated well into the recipe, then let it go. It would be best if you played with that a little bit. You can still bring the pan out and add further items every now and then: or test the cooking; all you have is to stop the unit.

How would you need air fryer?

The air fryer became famous primarily because of its various health effects. The comfort and convenience usage near the second area and this balance make it simple for anyone who prefers a balanced, tasty meal in a short amount of time.

To anyone who questions the functionality of air fryer and chooses traditional cooking methods, maybe the above facts would serve to persuade them to make a move to successful cooking. A considerable decrease in oil–cooking food in an air fryer takes no more than a tsp or two of the aluminum, but it still retains a certain quality. Quite cut short the usage of several cups of oil you'd like to prepare food in a microwave. The consequence is food which is not drenched in unnecessary fat that would choke the arteries.

Quick simply press-and-go action in this case–when preparing your food, will no matter how long have to check for your saucepan on the stove. That also implies no oil smudge and unpreventable injuries. In the cooking chamber, all the magic arises, just set your cooking requirements, click the right button and then let the air fryer do all the job.

Popping with spice-the food taste really emerges out in an air fryer. Given the small amount of oil that is used for cooking the food, the "fried" aroma is achieved. Washing is convenient–instead of with dishwasher-safe food containers, it's as easy and straightforward as physically removing and placing it in. One can quickly completely clean the cooking compartment with a rag and a gentle dishwashing soap.

Secure–Its components are food reliable, and the cooking method also allows to prevent accidents in the kitchen which can lead to oil burned.

The air fryer's structure seldom stays warm even though the voltage internally is at its height. Before handling such a kitchen gadget, the regular kitchen gloves should provide you with more than enough safety. Because precaution is better than cure.

The unparalleled versatile-this sophisticated device is much more than a fryer. You might also bake, grill, and roast in. A kind of mini conventional oven that is incredibly versatile than a fryer. Swift cooking times–Lower temperatures in the cooking chamber cut unique cooking times by half.

Because the temperature is retained during the cooking process, ensuring you don't need to bother regarding the current conduction overtaking the cooking. Such advantages end up making air fryers the perfect option available to safe cooking. No compromise on quality or versatility!

BREAKFAST:

Red Bell Peppers Salad

Preparation Time: 25 minutes
Servings: 4
Ingredients:
½ cup cheddar cheese; shredded
¼ cup coconut cream
1 cup red bell peppers; chopped.
2 tbsp. chives; chopped.
Cooking spray
A pinch of salt and black pepper
Directions:
Take a bowl and mix all the **Ingredients:** except the cooking spray and whisk well.
Pour the mix in a baking pan that fits the air fryer greased with cooking spray and place the pan in the machine
Cook at 360°F for 20 minutes, divide between plates and serve for breakfast.
Nutrition: Calories: 220; Fat: 14g; Fiber: 2g; Carbs: 5g; Protein: 11g

Cauliflower Rice Bowls

Preparation Time: 20 minutes
Servings: 4
Ingredients:
12 oz. cauliflower rice
1 lb. fresh spinach; torn
1 red bell pepper; chopped.
2 tbsp. olive oil
2 tbsp. lime juice
3 tbsp. stevia
Directions:
In your air fryer, mix all the **Ingredients:**, toss, cook at 370°F for 15 minutes, shaking halfway, divide between plates and serve for breakfast
Nutrition: Calories: 219; Fat: 14g; Fiber: 3g; Carbs: 5g; Protein: 7g

Avocado and Coconut Cream Bake

Preparation Time: 25 minutes
Servings: 4
Ingredients:
1 avocado, pitted; peeled and cubed
2 spring onions; chopped.
1 oz. parmesan cheese; grated
½ cup coconut cream
2 eggs; whisked
1 tbsp. olive oil
Salt and black pepper to taste.
Directions:
Take a bowl and mix the eggs with the rest of the **Ingredients:** except the oil and whisk well.
Grease a baking pan that fits the air fryer with the oil, pour the avocado mix, spread, put the pan in the machine and cook at 360°F for 20 minutes. Divide between plates and serve for breakfast
Nutrition: Calories: 271; Fat: 14g; Fiber: 3g; Carbs: 5g; Protein: 11g

Cheesy Spinach Muffins

Preparation Time: 20 minutes
Servings: 4
Ingredients:
2 eggs; whisked
1 ½ cups coconut milk
4 oz. baby spinach; chopped.
2 oz. parmesan cheese; grated
3 oz. almond flour
1 tbsp. baking powder
Cooking spray
Directions:
Take a bowl and mix all the **Ingredients:** except the cooking spray and whisk really well.
Grease a muffin pan that fits your air fryer with the cooking spray, divide the muffins mix
Introduce the pan in the air fryer, cook at 380°F for 15 minutes, divide between plates and serve.
Nutrition: Calories: 210; Fat: 12g; Fiber: 3g; Carbs: 5g; Protein: 8g

Celery and Bell Peppers

Preparation Time: 20 minutes
Servings: 4
Ingredients:
½ cup mozzarella cheese; shredded
1 celery stalk; chopped.
2 green onions; sliced
6 eggs; whisked
1 red bell pepper; roughly chopped.
2 tbsp. butter; melted
A pinch of salt and black pepper
Directions:
Take a bowl and mix all the **Ingredients:** except the butter and whisk well.
Preheat the air fryer at 360°F, add the butter, heat it up, add the celery and bell peppers mix and cook for 15 minutes, shaking the fryer once. Divide the mix between plates and serve for breakfast
Nutrition: Calories: 222; Fat: 12g; Fiber: 4g; Carbs: 5g; Protein: 7g

Spinach and Eggs

Preparation Time: 25 minutes
Servings: 4
Ingredients:
3 cups baby spinach
12 eggs; whisked
1 tbsp. olive oil
½ tsp. smoked paprika
Salt and black pepper to taste.
Directions:
Take a bowl and mix all the **Ingredients:** except the oil and whisk them well.
Heat up your air fryer at 360°F, add the oil, heat it up, add the eggs and spinach mix, cover, cook for 20 minutes, divide between plates and serve
Nutrition: Calories: 220; Fat: 11g; Fiber: 3g; Carbs: 4g; Protein: 6g

Red Cabbage Bowls

Preparation Time: 20 minutes
Servings: 4
Ingredients:
2 cups red cabbage; shredded
1 red bell pepper; sliced
1 small avocado, peeled, pitted and sliced
A drizzle of olive oil
Salt and black pepper to taste.
Directions:
Grease your air fryer with the oil, add all the **Ingredients:**, toss, cover and cook at 400°F for 15 minutes.
Divide into bowls and serve cold for breakfast
Nutrition: Calories: 209; Fat: 8g; Fiber: 2g; Carbs: 4g; Protein: 9g

Nuts Pudding

Preparation Time: 5 minutes
Cooking time: 20 minutes
Servings: 4
Ingredients:
1 cup coconut flakes, unsweetened and shredded
1 cup almonds, chopped
½ cup walnuts, chopped
½ cup maple syrup
2 cups almond milk
½ cup heavy cream
Directions:
In your air fryer's pan, combine the coconut flakes with the nuts and the other **Ingredients:**, toss and cook at 360 degrees F for 20 minutes.
Divide into bowls and serve for breakfast.
Nutrition: calories 201, fat 6, fiber 8, carbs 19, protein 6

Rice and Berries Pudding

Preparation Time: 5 minutes
Cooking time: 20 minutes
Servings: 4
Ingredients:
1 cup white rice
3 cups almond milk
1 cup blackberries
2 tablespoons sugar
2 tablespoons butter, soft
1 teaspoon vanilla extract
Directions:
In your air fryer's pan, combine the rice with the almond milk and the other **Ingredients:**, toss and cook at 370 degrees F for 20 minutes.
Divide the rice pudding into bowls and serve.
Nutrition: calories 202, fat 12, fiber 4, carbs 7, protein 2

Chicken Bowls

Preparation Time: 6 minutes
Cooking time: 20 minutes
Servings: 4
Ingredients:
8 eggs, whisked
1 pound chicken breast, skinless, boneless and cut into strips
1 tablespoon olive oil
1 yellow onion, chopped
1 teaspoon chili powder
1 cup baby spinach
1 tablespoon parsley, chopped
2 tablespoons chives, chopped
Salt and black pepper to the taste
Directions:
Heat up your air fryer with the oil at 360 degrees F, add the meat and onion and cook for 5 minutes.
Add the eggs mixed with the other **Ingredients:**, toss gently, cook for 15 minutes more, divide everything into bowls and serve for breakfast.
Nutrition: calories 251, fat 8, fiber 4, carbs 15, protein 4

Fennel and Eggs Mix

Preparation Time: 5 minutes
Cooking time: 20 minutes
Servings: 4
Ingredients:
1 tablespoon avocado oil
1 yellow onion, chopped
½ teaspoon cumin, ground
1 teaspoon rosemary, dried
8 eggs, whisked
1 fennel bulb, shredded
1 tablespoon chives, chopped
Salt and black pepper to the taste
Directions:
In a bowl, combine the onion with the eggs, fennel and the other **Ingredients:** except the oil and whisk.
Heat up your air fryer with the oil at 360 degrees F, add the oil, add the fennel mix, cover, cook for 20 minutes, divide between plates and serve for breakfast.
Nutrition: calories 220, fat 11, fiber 3, carbs 4, protein 6

Chives Salmon and Shrimp Bowls

Preparation Time: 5 minutes
Cooking time: 12 minutes
Servings: 4
Ingredients:
1 pound shrimp, peeled and deveined
½ pound salmon fillets, boneless and cubed
2 spring onions, chopped

2 teaspoons olive oil
1 cup baby kale
Salt and black pepper to the taste
1 tablespoon chives, chopped
Directions:
Preheat the air fryer with the oil at 330 degrees F, add the shrimp, salmon and the other **Ingredients:**, toss gently and cook for 12 minutes.
Divide everything into bowls and serve.
Nutrition: calories 244, fat 11, fiber 4, carbs 5, protein 7

Mozzarella Endives and Tomato Salad

Preparation Time: 5 minutes
Cooking time: 20 minutes
Servings: 4
Ingredients:
2 endives, shredded
½ pound cherry tomatoes, halved
1 tablespoon olive oil
4 eggs, whisked
Salt and black pepper to the taste
1 teaspoon sweet paprika
½ cup mozzarella, shredded
Directions:
Preheat the air fryer with the oil at 350 degrees F, add the tomatoes, endives and the other **Ingredients:** except the mozzarella and toss.
Sprinkle the mozzarella on top, cook for 20 minutes, divide into bowls and serve for breakfast.
Nutrition: calories 229, fat 13, fiber 3, carbs 4, protein 7

Green Beans and Olives

Preparation Time: 25 minutes
Servings: 2
Ingredients:
1 cup green beans; halved
4 eggs; whisked
2 spring onions; chopped.
¼ tsp. cumin, ground
Salt and black pepper to taste.
Directions:
Preheat the air fryer at 360°F, add all the **Ingredients:**, toss, cover, cook for 20 minutes, divide between plates and serve for breakfast
Nutrition: Calories: 183; Fat: 8g; Fiber: 2g; Carbs: 3g; Protein: 7g

Mixed Veggie Bake

Preparation Time: 25 minutes
Servings: 4
Ingredients:
2 garlic cloves; minced
7 oz. mozzarella; shredded
2 celery stalks; chopped.
½ cup white mushrooms; chopped.
½ cup red bell pepper; chopped.

1 tbsp. lemon juice
1 tsp. olive oil
1 tsp. oregano; dried
Salt and black pepper to taste.

Directions:

Preheat the Air Fryer at 350°F, add the oil and heat it up.

Add garlic, celery, mushrooms, bell pepper, salt, pepper, oregano, mozzarella and the lemon juice, toss and cook for 20 minutes. Divide between plates and serve for breakfast

Nutrition: Calories: 230; Fat: 11g; Fiber: 2g; Carbs: 4g; Protein: 6g

Poppy Seed Cake

Preparation Time: 24 minutes
Servings: 6
Ingredients:

1 cup blanched finely ground almond flour.
2 large eggs.
½ cup powdered erythritol
¼ cup unsalted butter; melted.
1 medium lemon.
¼ cup unsweetened almond milk
½ tsp. baking powder.
1 tsp. vanilla extract.
1 tsp. poppy seeds

Directions:

Take a large bowl, mix almond flour, erythritol, baking powder, butter, almond milk, eggs and vanilla.

Slice the lemon in half and squeeze the juice into a small bowl, then add to the batter

Using a fine grater, zest the lemon and add 1 tbsp. zest to the batter and stir. Add poppy seeds to batter.

Pour batter into nonstick 6-inch round cake pan. Place pan into the air fryer basket. Adjust the temperature to 300 Degrees F and set the timer for 14 minutes

When fully cooked, a toothpick inserted in center will come out mostly clean. The cake will finish cooking and firm up as it cools. Serve at room temperature.

Nutrition: Calories: 204; Protein: 3g; Fiber: 4g; Fat: 12g; Carbs: 19g

Asparagus Salad

Preparation Time: 15 minutes
Servings: 4
Ingredients:

1 cup baby arugula
1 bunch asparagus; trimmed
1 tbsp. balsamic vinegar
1 tbsp. cheddar cheese; grated
A pinch of salt and black pepper
Cooking spray

Directions:

Put the asparagus in your air fryer's basket, grease with cooking spray, season with salt and pepper and cook at 360°F for 10 minutes.

Take a bowl and mix the asparagus with the arugula and the vinegar, toss, divide between plates and serve hot with cheese sprinkled on top

Nutrition: Calories: 200; Fat: 5g; Fiber: 1g; Carbs: 4g; Protein: 5g

Eggplant and Chives Spread

Preparation Time: 25 minutes
Servings: 4
Ingredients:
3 eggplants
2 tbsp. olive oil
2 tbsp. chives; chopped.
2 tsp. sweet paprika
Salt and black pepper to taste.
Directions:
Put the eggplants in your air fryer's basket and cook them for 20 minutes at 380°F.
Peel the eggplants, put them in a blender, add the rest of the **Ingredients:**, pulse well
Divide into bowls and serve for breakfast.
Nutrition: Calories: 190; Fat: 7g; Fiber: 3g; Carbs: 5g; Protein: 3g

Tomatoes and Eggs

Preparation Time: 30 minutes
Servings: 4
Ingredients:
30 oz. canned tomatoes; chopped.
½ lb. cheddar; shredded
6 eggs; whisked
2 tbsp. olive oil
2 tbsp. chives; chopped.
Salt and black pepper to taste.
Directions:
Add the oil to your air fryer, heat it up at 350°F, add the tomatoes, eggs, salt and pepper and whisk.
Also add the cheese on top and sprinkle the chives on top
Cook for 25 minutes, divide between plates and serve.
Nutrition: Calories: 221; Fat: 8g; Fiber: 3g; Carbs: 4g; Protein: 8g

Hash Browns and Eggs Mix

Preparation Time: 10 minutes
Cooking time: 20 minutes
Servings: 4
Ingredients:
2 pounds hash browns
2 spring onions, chopped
2 bacon slices, chopped
1 tablespoon olive oil
1 green chili pepper, minced
4 eggs, whisked
Salt and black pepper to the taste
1 tablespoon chives, chopped
Directions:
Preheat the air fryer at 350 degrees F and add the oil.
Add the hash browns, spring onions and the other **Ingredients:** except the chives, stir well and cook at 360 degrees F for 20 minutes.
Divide the mix between plates and serve for breakfast.

Nutrition: calories 697, fat 33, fiber 5, carbs 86, protein 15

Ground Chicken and Eggs

Preparation Time: 5 minutes
Cooking time: 20 minutes
Servings: 4
Ingredients:
1 pound chicken breast, skinless, boneless and ground
1 tablespoon avocado oil
10 eggs, whisked
½ teaspoon rosemary, dried
1 teaspoon oregano, dried
1 tablespoon chives, chopped
Salt and black pepper to the taste
Directions:
Heat up your air fryer at 350 degrees F, add oil and heat it up.
Add the chicken, stir and cook for 5 minutes.
Add the eggs mixed with the other **Ingredients:**, toss everything and cook for 15 minutes.
Divide the mix between plates and serve.
Nutrition: calories 293, fat 13, fiber 4, carbs 4, protein 38

Spinach and Bacon Mix

Preparation Time: 5 minutes
Cooking time: 20 minutes
Servings: 4
Ingredients:
4 bacon slices, cubed
1 tablespoon olive oil
2 cups baby spinach
1 red bell pepper, chopped
1 green bell pepper, chopped
2 spring onions, chopped
4 eggs, whisked
1 cup cheddar cheese, shredded
Salt and black pepper to the taste
2 tablespoons chives, chopped
Directions:
Heat up your air fryer at 360 degrees F with the oil, add the peppers, spring onions and the bacon and cook for 5 minutes.
Add the eggs mixed with the other **Ingredients:**, toss everything and cook for 15 minutes more.
Divide the mix between plates and serve for breakfast.
Nutrition: calories 232, fat 15, fiber 4, carbs 4, protein 18

Salmon Burrito

Preparation Time: 5 minutes
Cooking time: 12 minutes
Servings: 4
Ingredients:
4 smoked salmon fillets, boneless, skinless and cut into strips
4 eggs, whisked
1 tomato, cubed

1 avocado, peeled, pitted and sliced
2 tablespoons salsa
1 tablespoon basil pesto
Salt and black pepper to the taste
½ cup cheddar cheese, shredded
4 corn tortillas

Directions:

In a bowl, mix the eggs with salt, pepper and the pesto, whisk, pour them in the air fryer's pan, put the pan in the air fryer's basket, cook for 6 minutes at 390 degrees and transfer the mix to a plate.

Arrange the tortillas on a working surface, divide the salmon, eggs, tomato and the remaining **Ingredients:** on each tortilla and roll them into burritos.

Line your air fryer with tin foil, add the burritos, cook them at 320 degrees F for 6 minutes more, divide between plates and serve for breakfast.

Nutrition: calories 280, fat 16, fiber 2, carbs 17, protein 17

Berries Oatmeal

Preparation Time: 5 minutes
Cooking time: 20 minutes
Servings: 4

Ingredients:

2 cups old fashioned oats
1/3 cup sugar
1 teaspoon vanilla extract
1 cup strawberries, halved
1 cup blueberries
2 cups almond milk
Cooking spray

Directions:

In a bowl, combine the oats with the sugar and the other **Ingredients:** and toss well.

Grease the air fryer with the cooking spray, heat it up at 330 degrees F, add the oats mix, cover and cook for 20 minutes.

Divide into bowls and serve for breakfast.

Nutrition: calories 687, fat 31, fiber 11, carbs 82, protein 13

Hash Browns and Tomatoes Mix

Preparation Time: 10 minutes
Cooking time: 30 minutes
Servings: 4

Ingredients:

2 pounds hash browns
4 eggs, whisked
1 pound cherry tomatoes, halved
2 tablespoons olive oil
1 red onion, chopped
2 spring onions, chopped
1 cup cheddar, shredded
2 tablespoons chives, chopped
Salt and black pepper to the taste

Directions:

Add the oil to your air fryer, heat it up at 350 degrees F, add the onion, spring onions and the tomatoes and cook for 5 minutes.
Add the hash browns and cook for 5 minutes more.
Add the remaining **Ingredients:**, whisk well everything, and cook for 20 minutes shaking the fryer halfway.
Divide everything between plates and serve for breakfast.
Nutrition: calories 807, fat 42, fiber 5, carbs 81, protein 27

Cheesy Eggs

Preparation Time: 10 minutes
Cooking time: 20 minutes
Servings: 4
Ingredients:
1 cup almond milk
12 eggs, whisked
1 tablespoon avocado oil
1 red bell pepper, chopped
1 green bell pepper, chopped
1 cup cream cheese
1 cup cheddar cheese, shredded
2 spring onions, chopped
Salt and black pepper to the taste
Directions:
Heat up your air fryer with the oil at 350 degrees F, add the bell peppers and cook for 2 minutes.
Add the eggs mixed with the remaining **Ingredients:**, toss everything and cook for 18 minutes more.
Divide everything between plates and serve.
Nutrition: calories 669, fat 56, fiber 5, carbs 15, protein 32

Basil Frittata

Preparation Time: 10 minutes
Cooking time: 20 minutes
Servings: 4
Ingredients:
2 tablespoons basil pesto
12 eggs, whisked
½ cup cheddar cheese, grated
2 tablespoons parsley, chopped
Salt and black pepper to the taste
2 tablespoons chives, chopped
6 tablespoons ricotta cheese
Cooking spray
Directions:
In a bowl, mix the eggs with the pesto and the other **Ingredients:** except the cooking spray and whisk well.
Grease the air fryer with the cooking sprat, heat it up at 320 degrees F, add the eggs mix, spread, and cook for 20 minutes.
Divide the frittata between plates and serve.
Nutrition: calories 280, fat 18, fiber 1, carbs 6, protein 29

Banana Cream Cheese Bowls

Preparation Time: 5 minutes
Cooking time: 20 minutes
Servings: 4
Ingredients:
2 cups almond milk
2 tablespoons brown sugar
½ cup cream cheese, soft
2 eggs, whisked
¼ teaspoon vanilla extract
2 bananas, peeled and chopped
1 cup coconut flakes, unsweetened
Cooking spray
Directions:
In a bowl, mix the almond milk with the cream cheese, sugar and the other **Ingredients:** except the cooking spray and whisk well.
Grease the air fryer with the cooking spray, heat it at 350 degrees F, add the banana mix, spread and cook for 20 minutes.
Divide into bowls and serve for breakfast.
Nutrition: calories 551, fat 49, fiber 6, carbs 26, protein 9

Paprika Potatoes and Sprouts

Preparation Time: 10 minutes
Cooking time: 10 minutes
Servings: 4
Ingredients:
4 eggs, whisked
2 sweet potatoes, peeled and cubed
1 tablespoon olive oil
2 spring onions, chopped
1 cup Brussels sprouts, trimmed and halved
Salt and black pepper to the taste
2 teaspoons sweet paprika
1 tablespoon chives, chopped
Directions:
Heat up your air fryer with the oil at 350 degrees F, add the spring onions, sprouts and the sweet potatoes and cook for 5 minutes.
Add the eggs and the remaining **Ingredients:**, toss and cook for 15 minutes more.
Divide the mix between plates and serve for breakfast right away.
Nutrition: calories 108, fat 1, fiber 4, carbs 5, protein 6

Mushroom Oats

Preparation Time: 5 minutes
Cooking time: 20 minutes
Servings: 4
Ingredients:
1 tablespoon avocado oil
2 spring onions, chopped
1 cup old fashioned oats
1 cup almond milk

2 eggs, whisked
6 white mushrooms, chopped
½ cup heavy cream
Salt and black pepper to the taste
¼ cup cheddar cheese, grated

Directions:

Heat up the air fryer with the oil at 360 degrees F, add the spring onions and the mushrooms and cook for 5 minutes.

Add the oats mixed with the milk and the other **Ingredients:**, toss and cook for 15 minutes more.

Divide the mix into bowls and serve for breakfast.

Nutrition: calories 419, fat 25, fiber 9, carbs 35, protein 12

Cheesy Cauliflower Mix

Preparation Time: 10 minutes
Cooking time: 20 minutes
Servings: 4

Ingredients:

1 pound cauliflower florets
4 eggs, whisked
½ cup heavy cream
1 cup cheddar cheese, shredded
2 teaspoons cilantro, chopped
1 tablespoon chives, chopped
Salt and black pepper to the taste

Directions:

Put the cauliflower in the air fryer, add the eggs mixed with the other **Ingredients:**, toss, cook at 350 degrees F for 20 minutes, divide between plates and serve for breakfast.

Nutrition: calories 194, fat 4, fiber 7, carbs 11, protein 6

Tomato and Pork Bake

Preparation Time: 5 minutes
Cooking time: 25 minutes
Servings: 4

Ingredients:

½ pound pork stew meat, cubed
1 cup tomatoes, cubed
1 tablespoon olive oil
1 teaspoon rosemary, dried
1 teaspoon turmeric powder
2 gold potatoes, peeled and cubed
1 cup cheddar cheese, grated
3 garlic cloves, minced
Salt and black pepper to the taste

Directions:

Heat up the air fryer with the oil at 360 degrees F, add the meat and brown for 5 minutes.

Add the tomatoes and the other **Ingredients:** except the cheese and toss.

Sprinkle the cheese on top, cook everything for 20 minutes, divide between plates and serve.

Nutrition: calories 187, fat 6, fiber 6, carbs 13, protein 5

Sausage and Zucchini Bake

Preparation Time: 5 minutes
Cooking time: 20 minutes
Servings: 4
Ingredients:
1 pound pork sausage, sliced
1 zucchini, sliced
1 red onion, chopped
1 tablespoon olive oil
1 cup mozzarella, shredded
4 eggs, whisked
1 tablespoon cilantro, chopped
1 teaspoon rosemary, dried
1 teaspoon cumin, ground
Salt and black pepper to the taste
Directions:
Heat up the air fryer with the oil at 360 degrees F, add the onion and the sausage and brown for 5 minutes.
Add the zucchini and the eggs mixed with the other **Ingredients:** except the cheese.
Sprinkle the cheese on top, cook the mix for 15 minutes more, divide between plates and serve for breakfast.
Nutrition: calories 270, fat 14, fiber 3, carbs 23, protein 16

Zucchini Frittata

Preparation Time: 10 minutes
Cooking time: 20 minutes
Servings: 4
Ingredients:
2 zucchinis, cubed
8 eggs, whisked
1 teaspoon sweet paprika
1 teaspoon rosemary, dried
1 red onion, chopped
Salt and black pepper to the taste
1 tablespoon butter, soft
Directions:
Grease the air fryer's pan with the butter and heat up the machine at 370 degrees F.
In a bowl, combine the zucchinis with the rest of the **Ingredients:**, whisk, pour into the pan and spread.
Cook for 20 minutes, slice and serve.
Nutrition: calories 170, fat 2, fiber 2, carbs 12, protein 4

Mushroom Hash

Preparation Time: 5 minutes
Cooking time: 20 minutes
Servings: 4
Ingredients:
1 pound white mushrooms, sliced
1 tablespoon avocado oil
1 red onion, chopped

1 teaspoon rosemary, dried
A pinch of salt and black pepper
1 cup cherry tomatoes, halved
4 eggs, whisked

Directions:

Heat up the air fryer with the oil at 370 degrees F, add the onion and the mushrooms and cook for 5 minutes.

Add the eggs mixed with the other **Ingredients:**, whisk everything and cook for 15 minutes more.

Divide everything between plates and serve for breakfast.

Nutrition: calories 170, fat 6, fiber 5, carbs 11, protein 2

Buttery Cheese Sandwich

Preparation Time: 10 minutes
Servings: 1
Ingredients:

2 tbsp butter
2 slices bread
3 slices American cheese

Directions:

Preheat the air fryer to 370 degrees F. Spread one tsp of butter on the outside of each of the bread slices. Place the cheese on the inside of one bread slice. Top with the other slice. Cook in the air fryer for 4 minutes. Flip the sandwich over and cook for an additional 4 minutes. Serve cut diagonally.

Olives & Tomato Tart with Feta Cheese

Preparation Time: 40 minutes
Servings: 2
Ingredients:

4 eggs
½ cup chopped tomatoes
1 cup crumbled feta cheese
1 tbsp chopped basil
1 tbsp chopped oregano
¼ cup chopped kalamata olives
¼ cup chopped onion
2 tbsp olive oil
½ cup milk
Salt and black pepper to taste

Directions:

Preheat the air fryer to 340 degrees F. Brush a pie pan with olive oil. Beat the eggs along with the milk and some salt and pepper. Stir in all of the remaining **Ingredients:**. Pour the egg mixture into the pan. Cook for 30 minutes.

Creamy Vanilla Berries Pastry

Preparation Time: 20 minutes
Servings: 3
Ingredients:

3 pastry dough sheets
2 tbsp mashed strawberries
2 tbsp mashed raspberries

¼ tsp vanilla extract
2 cups cream cheese
1 tbsp honey

Directions:

Preheat the air fryer to 375 degrees F. Divide the cream cheese between the dough sheets and spread it evenly. In a small bowl, combine the berries, honey and vanilla. Divide the mixture between the pastry sheets. Pinch the ends of the sheets, to form puff. Place the puffs on a lined baking dish. Place the dish in the air fryer and cook for 15 minutes.

Prosciutto & Salami Omelet

Preparation Time: 20 minutes
Servings: 2
Ingredients:

1 beef sausage, chopped
4 slices prosciutto, chopped
3 oz salami, chopped
1 cup grated mozzarella cheese
4 eggs
1 tbsp chopped onion
1 tbsp ketchup

Directions:

Preheat the air fryer to 350 degrees F. Whisk the eggs with the ketchup, in a bowl. Stir in the onion. Brown the sausage in the air fryer for 2 minutes. Meanwhile, combine the egg mixture, mozzarella cheese, salami and prosciutto. Pour the egg mixture over the sausage and give it a stir. Cook for 10 minutes.

Hazelnut Bread Pudding with Honey & Raisins

Preparation Time: 45 minutes
Servings: 3
Ingredients:

8 slices of bread
½ cup buttermilk
¼ cup honey
1 cup milk
2 eggs
½ tsp vanilla extract
2 tbsp butter, softened
¼ cup sugar
4 tbsp raisins
2 tbsp chopped hazelnuts
Cinnamon for garnish

Directions:

Preheat the air fryer to 310 degrees F. Beat the eggs along with the buttermilk, honey, milk, vanilla, sugar and butter. Stir in raisins and hazelnuts. Cut the bread into cubes and place them, in a bowl. Pour the milk mixture over the bread. Let soak for 10 minutes. Cook the bread pudding for 30 minutes and garnish with cinnamon.

Speedy Bacon & Egg Sandwich

Preparation Time: 10 minutes
Servings: 1
Ingredients:
1 whole egg, cracked
1 slice English bacon
Salt and black pepper to taste
1 slice bread
½ cup butter
Directions:
Preheat your Air Fryer to 400 degrees F. Spread butter on one side of the bread slice. Add the cracked egg on top and season with salt and pepper. Place bacon on top. Arrange the bread slice in your Air Fryer's cooking basket and cook for 3-5 minutes. Serve and enjoy!

Parmesan Sausage Frittata with Tomatoes

Preparation Time: 15 minutes
Servings: 1
Ingredients:
½ sausage, chopped
Salt and black pepper to taste
A bunch of parsley, chopped
3 whole eggs
1 tbsp olive oil
1 slice bread
4 cherry tomatoes, halved
1 slice bread
2 tbsp parmesan, shredded for garnish
Directions:
Preheat your Air Fryer to 360 degrees F. Place tomatoes and sausages in your air fryer's cooking basket and cook for 5 minutes. In a bowl, mix baked tomatoes, sausages, eggs, salt, parsley, parmesan, oil and pepper.
Add the bread to the air fryer cooking basket and cook for 5 minutes. Add the frittata mixture over baked bread and top with parmesan. Serve and enjoy!

Cheesy Berry-Flavored French Toast

Preparation Time: 15 minutes
Servings: 4
Ingredients:
2 eggs, beaten
4 slices bread
3 tbsp sugar
1 ½ cups corn flakes
⅓ cup milk
¼ tsp nutmeg
4 tbsp berry-flavored cheese
¼ tsp salt
Directions:
Preheat your Air Fryer to 400 degrees F. In a bowl, mix sugar, eggs, nutmeg, salt and milk. In a separate bowl, mix blueberries and cheese. Take 2 bread slices and pour the blueberry mixture over the slices.

Top with the milk mixture. Cover with the remaining two slices to make sandwiches. Dredge the sandwiches over cornflakes to coat well. Lay the sandwiches in your air fryer's cooking basket and cook for 8 minutes. Serve with berries and syrup.

Peppery Tofu & Green Onion Omelet with Soy Sauce

Preparation Time: 20 minutes
Servings: 1
Ingredients:
1 small Japanese tofu, cubed
3 whole eggs
Pepper to taste
1 tsp coriander
1 tsp cumin
2 tbsp soy sauce
2 tbsp green onion, chopped
Olive oil
1 whole onion, chopped
Directions:
In a bowl, mix eggs, soy sauce, cumin, pepper, oil, and salt. Add cubed tofu to baking forms and pour the egg mixture on top. Place the prepared forms in the air fryer cooking basket and cook for 10 minutes at 400 F. Serve with a sprinkle of coriander and green onion.

Cinnamon Pineapples Grilled with Honey

Preparation Time: 15 minutes
Servings: 2
Ingredients:
1 tsp cinnamon
5 pineapple slices
½ cup brown sugar
1 tbsp basil, chopped for garnish
1 tbsp honey, for garnish
Directions:
Preheat your air fryer to 340 degrees F. In a small bowl, mix brown sugar and cinnamon. Drizzle the sugar mixture over your pineapple slices and set aside for 20 minutes.
Place the pineapple rings in the air fryer cooking basket and cook for 10 minutes. Flip the pineapples and cook for 10 minutes more. Serve with basil and a drizzle of honey.

Creamy Beacon & Thyme Omelet Cups

Preparation Time: 25 minutes
Servings: 4
Ingredients:
4 crusty rolls
5 eggs, beaten
A pinch of salt
½ tsp thyme, dried
3 strips precooked bacon, chopped
2 tbsp heavy cream
4 Gouda cheese mini wedges, thin slices

Directions:
Preheat your air fryer 330 degrees F. Cut the tops off the rolls and remove the inside with your fingers. Line the rolls with a slice of cheese and press down, so the cheese conforms to the inside of the roll. In a bowl, mix eggs with heavy cream, bacon, thyme, salt and pepper.
Stuff the rolls with the egg mixture. Lay the rolls in your air fryer's cooking basket and bake for 8 to 12 minutes or until the eggs become puffy and the roll shows a golden brown texture.

Easy Murshroom & Turkey Sandwich

Preparation Time: 15 minutes
Servings: 1
Ingredients:
⅓ cup shredded leftover turkey
⅓ cup sliced mushrooms
1 tbsp butter, divided
2 tomato slices
½ tsp red pepper flakes
¼ tsp salt
¼ tsp black pepper
1 hamburger bun
Directions:
Melt half of the butter and add the mushrooms. Cook for 4 minutes. Meanwhile, cut the bun in half and spread the remaining butter on the outside of the bun. Place the turkey on one half of the bun.
Arrange the mushroom slices on top of the turkey. Place the tomato slices on top of the mushrooms. Sprinkle with salt pepper and red pepper flakes. Top with the other bun half. Cook for 5 minutes at 350 F.

Cheesy Bacon & Turkey Calzone

Preparation Time: 20 minutes
Servings: 4
Ingredients:
Pizza dough
4 oz cheddar cheese, grated
1 oz mozzarella cheese
1 oz bacon, diced
2 cups cooked and shredded turkey
1 egg, beaten
1 tsp thyme
4 tbsp tomato paste
1 tsp basil
1 tsp oregano
Salt and black pepper to taste
Directions:
Preheat the air fryer to 350 degrees F. Divide the pizza dough into 4 equal pieces so you have the dough for 4 small pizza crusts. Combine the tomato paste, basil, oregano, and thyme, in a small bowl.
Brush the mixture onto the crusts just make sure not to go all the way and avoid brushing near the edges on one half of each crust, place ½ turkey, and season the meat with some salt and pepper.

Top the meat with some bacon. Combine the cheddar and mozzarella and divide it between the pizzas, making sure that you layer only one half of the dough. Brush the edges of the crust with the beaten egg. Fold the crust and seal with a fork. Cook for 10 minutes.

Salty Parsnip Hash Browns

Preparation Time: 20 minutes
Servings: 2
Ingredients:
1 large parsnip, grated
3 eggs, beaten
½ tsp garlic powder
¼ tsp nutmeg
1 tbsp olive oil
1 cup flour
Salt and black pepper to taste
Directions:
Heat olive oil in the air fryer at 390 degrees F. In a bowl, combine flour, eggs, parsnip, nutmeg, and garlic powder. Season with salt and pepper. Form patties out of the mixture. Arrange in the air fryer and cook for 15 minutes.

Creamy Bacon & Egg Wraps with Spicy Salsa

Preparation Time: 15 minutes
Servings: 3
Ingredients:
3 tortillas
2 previously scrambled eggs
3 slices bacon, cut into strips
3 tbsp salsa
3 tbsp cream cheese, divided
1 cup grated pepper Jack cheese
Directions:
Preheat the air fryer to 390 degrees F. Spread one tbsp. of cream cheese onto each tortilla. Divide the eggs and bacon between the tortillas evenly. Top with salsa. Sprinkle some grated cheese over. Roll up the tortillas. Cook for 10 minutes.

Sweet Strawberries Pancake

Preparation Time: 30 minutes
Servings: 4
Ingredients:
3 eggs, beaten
2 tbsp unsalted butter
½ cup flour
2 tbsp sugar, powdered
½ cup milk
1½ cups fresh strawberries, sliced
Directions:
Preheat your Air Fryer to 330 degrees F. Add butter to a pan and melt over low heat. In a bowl, mix flour, milk, eggs and vanilla until fully incorporated. Add the mixture to the pan with melted butter.

Place the pan in your air fryer's cooking basket and cook for 12-16 minutes until the pancake is fluffy and golden brown. Drizzle powdered sugar and toss sliced strawberries on top.

Spinach & Kale Balsamic Chicken

Preparation Time: 20 minutes
Servings: 1
Ingredients:
½ cup baby spinach leaves
½ cup shredded romaine
3 large kale leaves, chopped
4 oz chicken breasts, cut into cubes
3 tbsp olive oil, divided
1 tsp balsamic vinegar
1 garlic clove, minced
Salt and black pepper to taste
Directions:
Place the chicken, 1 tbsp. olive oil and garlic, in a bowl. Season with salt and pepper and toss to combine.
Put on a lined baking dish and cook for 14 minutes at 390F. Meanwhile, place the greens in a large bowl. Add the remaining olive oil and balsamic vinegar. Season with salt and pepper and toss to combine. Top with the chicken.

Creamy Parmesan & Ham Shirred Eggs

Preparation Time: 20 minutes
Servings: 2
Ingredients:
2 tsp butter, for greasing
4 eggs, divided
2 tbsp heavy cream
4 slices of ham
3 tbsp Parmesan cheese
¼ tsp paprika
¾ tsp salt
¼ tsp pepper
2 tsp chopped chives
Directions:
Preheat the air fryer to 320 degrees F. Grease a pie pan with the butter. Arrange the ham slices on the bottom of the pan to cover it completely. Whisk one egg along with the heavy cream, salt and pepper, in a small bowl.
Pour the mixture over the ham slices. Crack the other eggs over the ham. Sprinkle with Parmesan cheese. Cook for 14 minutes. Season with paprika, garnish with chives and serve with bread.

Quick Paprika Eggs

Preparation Time: 15 minutes
Servings: 6
Ingredients:
6 large eggs
1 tsp paprika
Directions:
Preheat your air fryer 300 degrees F. Lay the eggs in your air fryer's basket and bake for at least 8 minutes for a slightly runny yolk or 12 to 15 minutes for a firmer yolk. Using tongs, place the eggs in a bowl with icy water. Allow to cool in cold water for 5 minutes before cracking the shell under water. Serve sprinkled with paprika.

Classic Cheddar Cheese Omelet

Preparation Time: 15 minutes
Servings: 1
Ingredients:
2 eggs, beaten
Black pepper to taste
1 cup cheddar cheese, shredded
1 whole onion, chopped
2 tbsp soy sauce
Directions:
Preheat your Air Fryer to 340 degrees F. Drizzle soy sauce over the chopped onions. Place the onions in your air fryer's cooking basket and cook for 8 minutes. In a bowl, mix the beaten eggs with salt and pepper.
Pour the egg mixture over onions (in the cooking basketand cook for 3 minutes. Add cheddar cheese over eggs and bake for 2 more minutes. Serve and enjoy!

Buttered Apple & Brie Cheese Sandwich

Preparation Time: 8 - 10 minutes
Servings: 1
Ingredients:
2 bread slices
½ apple, thinly sliced
2 tsp butter
2 oz brie cheese, thinly sliced
Directions:
Spread butter on the outside of the bread slices. Arrange apple slices on the inside of one bread slice. Place brie slices on top of the apple. Top with the other slice of bread. Cook for 5 minutes at 350 F. Serve cut diagonally.

Fresh Kale & Cottage Omelet

Preparation Time: 15 minutes
Servings: 1
Ingredients:
3 eggs
3 tbsp cottage cheese
3 tbsp chopped kale
½ tbsp chopped basil
½ tbsp chopped parsley
Salt and black pepper to taste
1 tsp olive oil
Directions:
Heat oil at 330 F. Beat the eggs with salt and pepper, in a bowl. Stir in the rest of the **Ingredients:**. Pour the mixture into the air fryer and cook for 10 minutes, until slightly golden and set.

Vanilla & Cinnamon Toast Toppet

Preparation Time: 10 minutes
Servings: 6
Ingredients:
12 slices bread
½ cup sugar

1 ½ tsp cinnamon
1 stick of butter, softened
1 tsp vanilla extract
Directions:
Preheat the air fryer to 400 degrees F. Combine all **Ingredients:**, except the bread, in a bowl. Spread the buttery cinnamon mixture onto the bread slices. Place the bread slices in the air fryer. Cook for 5 minutes.

Parsley Onion & Feta Tart

Preparation Time: 30 minutes
Servings: 3
Ingredients:
3½ pounds Feta cheese
Black pepper to taste
1 whole onion, chopped
2 tbsp parsley, chopped
1 egg yolk
Olive oil for drizzling
5 sheets frozen filo pastry
Directions:
Cut each of the 5 filo sheets into three equal sized strips. Cover the strips with oil. In a bowl, mix onion, pepper, feta, salt, egg yolk, and parsley.
Make triangles using the cut strips and add a little bit of the feta mixture on top of each triangle. Place the triangles in fryer's basket and cook for 3 minutes at 400 F. Serve with a drizzle of oil and green onions.

Tomato, Basil & Mozzarella Breakfast

Preparation Time: 7 minutes
Servings: 1
Ingredients:
2 slices of bread
4 tomato slices
4 mozzarella slices
1 tbsp olive oil
1 tbsp chopped basil
Salt and black pepper to taste
Directions:
Preheat the air fryer to 370 degrees F. Place the bread slices in the air fryer and toast for 3 minutes. Arrange two tomato slices on each bread slice. Season with salt and pepper.
Top each slice with 2 mozzarella slices. Return to the air fryer and cook for 1 minute more. Drizzle the caprese toasts with olive oil and top with chopped basil.

Cinnamon-Orange Toast

Preparation Time: 15 minutes
Servings: 6
Ingredients:
12 slices bread
½ cup sugar
1 stick butter
1½ tbsp vanilla extract
1½ tbsp cinnamon

2 oranges, zested

Directions:

In a microwave proof bowl, mix butter, sugar and vanilla extract. Warm and stir the mixture for 30 seconds until everything melts. Add in orange zest. Pour the mixture over bread slices. Lay the bread slices in your air fryer's cooking basket and cook for 5 minutes at 400 F. Serve with fresh banana and berry sauce.

Herby Parmesan Bagel

Preparation Time: 6 minutes
Servings: 1
Ingredients:

2 tbsp butter, softened
1 tsp dried basil
1 tsp dried parsley
1 tsp garlic powder
1 tbsp Parmesan cheese
Salt and black pepper to taste
1 bagel

Directions:

Preheat the air fryer to 370 degrees. Cut the bagel in half. Place in the air fryer and cook for 3 minutes. Combine the butter, Parmesan, garlic, basil, and parsley in a small bowl. Season with salt and pepper, to taste. Spread the mixture onto the toasted bagel. Return the bagel to the air fryer and cook for an additional 3 minutes.

Porridge with Honey & peanut Butter

Preparation Time: 5 minutes
Servings: 4
Ingredients:

2 cups steel cut oats
1 cup flax seeds
1 tbsp peanut butter
1 tbsp butter
4 cups milk
4 tbsp honey

Directions:

Preheat the air fryer to 390 degrees F. Combine all of the **Ingredients:** in an ovenproof bowl. Place in the air fryer and cook for 5 minutes. Stir and serve.

Classic Bacon & Egg English Muffin

Preparation Time: 10 minutes
Servings: 1
Ingredients:

1 egg
1 English muffin
2 slices of bacon
Salt and black pepper to taste

Directions:

Preheat the air fryer to 395 F. Crack the egg into a ramekin. Place the muffin, egg and bacon in the air fryer. Cook for 6 minutes. Let cool slightly so you can assemble the sandwich. Cut the muffin in half. Place the egg on one half and season with salt and pepper. Arrange the bacon on top. Top with the other muffin half.

Almond Chicken Bake

Preparation Time: 25 minutes
Servings: 4
Ingredients:
1 cup chicken meat, cooked and shredded
½ cup almond milk
¼ cup almonds; chopped.
4 eggs; whisked
½ tsp. oregano; dried
Cooking spray
Salt and black pepper to taste.
Directions:
Take a bowl and mix the eggs with the rest of the **Ingredients:** except the cooking spray and whisk well.
Grease a baking pan with the cooking spray, pour the chicken mix into the pan, put the pan in the machine and cook the omelet at 350°F for 25 minutes. Divide between plates and serve for breakfast
Nutrition: Calories: 216; Fat: 11g; Fiber: 3g; Carbs: 5g; Protein: 9g

Broccoli and Cheddar Bake

Preparation Time: 25 minutes
Servings: 4
Ingredients:
1 broccoli head, florets separated and roughly chopped.
4 eggs; whisked
1 cup almond milk
2 oz. cheddar cheese; grated
2 tsp. cilantro; chopped.
Salt and black pepper to taste.
Directions:
Take a bowl and mix the eggs with the milk, cilantro, salt and pepper and whisk.
Put the broccoli in your air fryer, add the eggs mix over it, spread, sprinkle the cheese on top, cook at 350°F for 25 minutes, divide between plates and serve
Nutrition: Calories: 214; Fat: 14g; Fiber: 2g; Carbs: 4g; Protein: 9g

Egg, Bacon and Cheese Roll Ups

Preparation Time: 30 minutes
Servings: 4
Ingredients:
12 slices sugar-free bacon.
½ medium green bell pepper; seeded and chopped
6 large eggs.
¼ cup chopped onion
1 cup shredded sharp Cheddar cheese.
½ cup mild salsa, for dipping
2 tbsp. unsalted butter.
Directions:
In a medium skillet over medium heat, melt butter. Add onion and pepper to the skillet and sauté until fragrant and onions are translucent, about 3 minutes

Whisk eggs in a small bowl and pour into skillet. Scramble eggs with onions and peppers until fluffy and fully cooked, about 5 minutes. Remove from heat and set aside

On work surface, place three slices of bacon side by side, overlapping about ¼-inch. Place ¼ cup scrambled eggs in a heap on the side closest to you and sprinkle ¼ cup cheese on top of the eggs. Tightly roll the bacon around the eggs and secure the seam with a toothpick if necessary. Place each roll into the air fryer basket

Adjust the temperature to 350 Degrees F and set the timer for 15 minutes. Rotate the rolls halfway through the cooking time. Bacon will be brown and crispy when completely cooked. Serve immediately with salsa for dipping.

Nutrition: Calories: 460; Protein: 22g; Fiber: 8g; Fat: 37g; Carbs: 1g

Zucchini and Watercress Salad

Preparation Time: 19 minutes

Servings: 2

Ingredients:

2 cups zucchini, roughly cubed

1 cup parmesan cheese; grated

1 cup watercress; torn

1 tbsp. olive oil

Cooking spray

Directions:

Now, take a pan that fits in your air fryer and grease it with the cooking spray, add all the **Ingredients:** except the cheese, sprinkle the cheese on top and cook at 390°F for 15 minutes Divide into bowls and serve for breakfast.

Nutrition: Calories: 202; Fat: 11g; Fiber: 3g; Carbs: 5g; Protein: 4g

Bell Peppers and Eggs

Preparation Time: 25 minutes

Servings: 4

Ingredients:

1 orange bell pepper; cut into strips

4 eggs; whisked

1 red bell pepper; cut into strips

1 green bell pepper; cut into strips

2 tbsp. mozzarella; shredded

Cooking spray

Salt and black pepper to taste.

Directions:

Take a bowl and mix the eggs with all the bell peppers, salt and pepper and toss.

Preheat the air fryer at 350°F, grease it with cooking spray, pour the eggs mixture, spread well, sprinkle the mozzarella on top and cook for 20 minutes. Divide between plates and serve for breakfast

Nutrition: Calories: 229; Fat: 13g; Fiber: 3g; Carbs: 4g; Protein: 7g

Hard-Boiled Eggs

Preparation Time: 20 minutes

Servings: 4

Ingredients:

1 cup water

4 large eggs.

Directions:
Place eggs into a 4-cup round baking-safe dish and pour water over eggs. Place dish into the air fryer basket.
Adjust the temperature to 300 Degrees F and set the timer for 18 minutes. Store cooked eggs in the refrigerator until ready to use or peel and eat warm.
Nutrition: Calories: 77; Protein: 3g; Fiber: 0g; Fat: 4g; Carbs: 6g

POULTRY

Buffalo Chicken Tenders

Preparation Time: 35 minutes
Servings: 4
Ingredients:
1 lb. boneless, skinless chicken tenders
1 ½ oz. pork rinds, finely ground
¼ cup hot sauce
1 tsp. garlic powder.
1 tsp. chili powder
Directions:
Place chicken tenders in large bowl and pour hot sauce over them. Toss tenders in hot sauce, evenly coating.
In a separate large bowl, mix ground pork rinds with chili powder and garlic powder
Place each tender in the ground pork rinds, covering completely.
Wet your hands with water and press down the pork rinds into the chicken
Place the tenders in a single layer into the air fryer basket. Adjust the temperature to 375 Degrees F and set the timer for 20 minutes. Serve warm.
Nutrition: Calories: 160; Protein: 23g; Fiber: 4g; Fat: 4g; Carbs: 0g

Turmeric Chicken Wings

Preparation Time: 35 minutes
Servings: 4
Ingredients:
2 lb. chicken wings; halved
4 garlic cloves; minced
¼ cup red vinegar
1 tbsp. garlic powder
4 tbsp. olive oil
1 tsp. turmeric powder
Salt and black pepper to taste.
Directions:
Take a bowl and mix the chicken with all the other **Ingredients:** and toss well
Put the chicken wings in your air fryer's basket and cook at 370°F for 30 minutes, flipping the meat halfway.
Divide everything between plates and serve with a side salad.
Nutrition: Calories: 250; Fat: 12g; Fiber: 4g; Carbs: 6g; Protein: 15g

Almond Chicken

Preparation Time: 40 minutes
Servings: 4
Ingredients:
2 (6-oz.boneless, skinless chicken breasts
¼ cup slivered almonds
1 tbsp. Dijon mustard
2 tbsp. full-fat mayonnaise
Directions:
Pulse the almonds in a food processor or chop until finely chopped. Place almonds evenly on a plate and set aside. Completely slice each chicken breast in half lengthwise.

Mix the mayonnaise and mustard in a small bowl and then coat chicken with the mixture
Lay each piece of chicken in the chopped almonds to fully coat. Carefully move the pieces into the air fryer basket
Adjust the temperature to 350 Degrees F and set the timer for 25 minutes. Chicken will be done when it has reached an internal temperature of 165 Degrees F or more. Serve warm.
Nutrition: Calories: 195; Protein: 29g; Fiber: 8g; Fat: 11g; Carbs: 8g

Cinnamon Duck Breasts

Preparation Time: 25 minutes
Servings: 2
Ingredients:
2 duck breasts; boneless and skin scored
4 tbsp. stevia
3 tbsp. balsamic vinegar
¼ tsp. cinnamon powder
A pinch of salt and black pepper
Directions:
Take a bowl and mix the duck breasts with the rest of the **Ingredients:** and rub well.
Put the duck breasts in your air fryer's basket and cook at 380°F for 10 minutes on each side. Divide everything between plates and serve
Nutrition: Calories: 294; Fat: 12g; Fiber: 4g; Carbs: 6g; Protein: 15g

Mediterranean Chicken

Preparation Time: 40 minutes
Servings: 4
Ingredients:
1 lb. chicken thighs; boneless and skinless
½ lb. asparagus, trimmed and halved
1 zucchini; halved lengthwise and sliced into half-moons
3 garlic cloves; minced
Juice of 1 lemon
2 tbsp. olive oil
1 tsp. oregano; dried
A pinch of salt and black pepper
Directions:
Take a bowl and mix the chicken with all the **Ingredients:** except the asparagus and the zucchinis, toss and leave aside for 15 minutes
Add the zucchinis and the asparagus, toss, put everything into a pan that fits the air fryer and cook at 380°F for 25 minutes. Divide everything between plates and serve.
Nutrition: Calories: 280; Fat: 11g; Fiber: 4g; Carbs: 6g; Protein: 17g

Ginger Chicken Breasts

Preparation Time: 25 minutes
Servings: 4
Ingredients:
4 chicken breasts, skinless; boneless and halved
¼ cup chicken stock
2 tbsp. stevia
1 tbsp. ginger, grated
4 tbsp. coconut aminos
1 tsp. olive oil

Salt and black pepper to taste.
Directions:
In a pan that fits the air fryer, combine the chicken with the ginger and all the **Ingredients:** and toss.
Put the pan in your air fryer and cook at 4380°F for 20, shaking the fryer halfway
Divide between plates and serve with a side salad.
Nutrition: Calories: 256; Fat: 12g; Fiber: 4g; Carbs: 6g; Protein: 14g

Chicken Patties

Preparation Time: 27 minutes
Servings: 4
Ingredients:
1 lb. ground chicken thigh meat
2 oz. pork rinds, finely ground
½ cup shredded mozzarella cheese
1 large egg.
¼ tsp. onion powder.
½ tsp. garlic powder.
1 tsp. dried parsley.
Directions:
Take a large bowl, mix ground chicken, mozzarella, parsley, garlic powder and onion powder. Form into four patties.
Place patties in the freezer for 15–20 minutes until they begin to firm up.
Whisk egg in a medium bowl. Place the ground pork rinds into a large bowl
Dip each chicken patty into the egg and then press into pork rinds to fully coat. Place patties into the air fryer basket
Adjust the temperature to 360 Degrees F and set the timer for 12 minutes.
Patties will be firm and cooked to an internal temperature of 165 Degrees F when done. Serve immediately.
Nutrition: Calories: 304; Protein: 37g; Fiber: 1g; Fat: 14g; Carbs: 9g

Crispy Chicken Wings

Preparation Time: 35 minutes
Servings: 4
Ingredients:
2 lb. chicken wings
¼ cup olive oil
Zest of 1 lemon, grated
2 garlic cloves; minced
Juice of 2 lemons
A pinch of salt and black pepper
Directions:
Take a bowl and mix the chicken wings with the rest of the **Ingredients:** and toss well
Put the chicken wings in your air fryer's basket and cook at 400°F for 30 minutes, shaking halfway. Divide between plates and serve with a side salad
Nutrition: Calories: 263; Fat: 14g; Fiber: 4g; Carbs: 6g; Protein: 15g

Chives Chicken Tenders

Preparation Time: 25 minutes
Servings: 4
Ingredients:
1 lb. chicken tenders, boneless, skinless
1 tbsp. chives; chopped
A drizzle of olive oil
Juice of 1 lemon
A pinch of salt and black pepper
Directions:
Take a bowl and mix the chicken tenders with all **Ingredients:** except the chives, toss, put the meat in your air fryer's basket and cook at 370°F for 10 minutes on each side
Divide between plates and serve with chives sprinkled on top.
Nutrition: Calories: 230; Fat: 13g; Fiber: 4g; Carbs: 6g; Protein: 16g

Fajita Chicken Breast

Preparation Time: 35 minutes
Servings: 4
Ingredients:
2 (6-oz.boneless, skinless chicken breasts
1 medium green bell pepper; seeded and sliced
¼ medium white onion; peeled. And sliced
1 tbsp. coconut oil
1 tsp. ground cumin
½ tsp. garlic powder.
2 tsp. chili powder
Directions:
Slice each chicken breast completely in half lengthwise into two even pieces. Using a meat tenderizer, lb. out the chicken until it's about ¼-inch thickness
Lay each slice of chicken out and place three slices of onion and four slices of green pepper on the end closest to you. Begin rolling the peppers and onions tightly into the chicken. Secure the roll with either toothpicks or a couple pieces of butcher's twine
Drizzle coconut oil over chicken. Sprinkle each side with chili powder, cumin and garlic powder. Place each roll into the air fryer basket. Adjust the temperature to 350 Degrees F and set the timer for 25 minutes. Serve warm.
Nutrition: Calories: 146; Protein: 18g; Fiber: 2g; Fat: 9g; Carbs: 2g

Jalapeño Popper Hasselback Chicken

Preparation Time: 40 minutes
Servings: 2
Ingredients:
4 slices sugar-free bacon; cooked and crumbled
2 (6-oz.boneless, skinless chicken breasts
2 oz. full-fat cream cheese; softened.
¼ cup sliced pickled jalapeños
½ cup shredded sharp Cheddar cheese, divided.
Directions:
Take a medium bowl, place cooked bacon, then fold in cream cheese, half of the Cheddar and the jalapeño slices.

Use a sharp knife to make slits in each of the chicken breasts about ¾of the way across the chicken, being careful not to cut all the way through. Depending on the size of the chicken breast, you'll likely have 6–8 slits per breast

Spoon the cream cheese mixture into the slits of the chicken. Sprinkle remaining shredded cheese over chicken breasts and place into the air fryer basket. Adjust the temperature to 350 Degrees F and set the timer for 20 minutes. Serve warm.

Nutrition: Calories: 501; Protein: 58g; Fiber: 2g; Fat: 23g; Carbs: 6g

Chicken and Pepperoni Pizza Bake

Preparation Time: 25 minutes

Servings: 4

Ingredients:

20 slices pepperoni

2 cups cubed cooked chicken

1 cup shredded mozzarella cheese

¼ cup grated Parmesan cheese.

1 cup low-carb, sugar-free pizza sauce

Directions:

In a 4-cup round baking dish add chicken, pepperoni and pizza sauce. Stir so meat is completely covered with sauce.

Top with mozzarella and grated Parmesan. Place dish into the air fryer basket. Adjust the temperature to 375 Degrees F and set the timer for 15 minutes

Dish will be brown and bubbling when cooked. Serve immediately.

Nutrition: Calories: 353; Protein: 34g; Fiber: 0g; Fat: 14g; Carbs: 5g

Spring Chicken

Preparation Time: 30 minutes

Servings: 4

Ingredients:

4 chicken breasts, skinless; boneless and halved

4 tomatoes; cut into wedges

2 yellow bell peppers; cut into wedges

2 zucchinis; sliced

2 tbsp. olive oil

1 tsp. Italian seasoning

Directions:

In a baking dish that fits your air fryer, mix all the **Ingredients:**, toss, introduce in the fryer and cook at 380°F for 25 minutes.

Divide everything between plates and serve.

Nutrition: Calories: 280; Fat: 12g; Fiber: 4g; Carbs: 6g; Protein: 14g

Chicken Fajitas

Preparation Time: 25 minutes

Servings: 2

Ingredients:

10 oz. boneless, skinless chicken breast, sliced into ¼-inch strips

½ medium red bell pepper; seeded and sliced

¼ medium onion; peeled.and sliced

½ medium green bell pepper; seeded and sliced

1 tbsp. chili powder

2 tbsp. coconut oil; melted

½ tsp. paprika
½ tsp. garlic powder.
½ tsp. cumin

Directions:

Place chicken and coconut oil into a large bowl and sprinkle with chili powder, cumin, paprika and garlic powder. Toss chicken until well coated with seasoning. Place chicken into the air fryer basket. Adjust the temperature to 350 Degrees F and set the timer for 15 minutes

Add onion and peppers into the fryer basket when the timer has 7 minutes remaining

Toss the chicken two or three times during cooking. Vegetables should be tender and chicken fully cooked to at least 165 Degrees F internal temperature when finished. Serve warm.

Nutrition: Calories: 326; Protein: 35g; Fiber: 2g; Fat: 19g; Carbs: 4g

Chicken Enchiladas

Preparation Time: 30 minutes
Servings: 4
Ingredients:

½ lb. medium-sliced deli chicken
1 medium avocado; peeled, pitted and sliced
1 cup shredded medium Cheddar cheese.
½ cup shredded Monterey jack cheese
⅓ cup low-carb enchilada sauce, divided.
½ cup full-fat sour cream.
1 ½ cups shredded cooked chicken

Directions:

Take a large bowl, mix shredded chicken and half of the enchilada sauce. Lay slices of deli chicken on a work surface and spoon 2 tbsp. shredded chicken mixture onto each slice

Sprinkle 2 tbsp. of Cheddar onto each roll. Gently roll closed

In a 4-cup round baking dish, place each roll, seam side down. Pour remaining sauce over rolls and top with Monterey jack. Place dish into the air fryer basket. Adjust the temperature to 370 Degrees F and set the timer for 10 minutes.

Enchiladas will be golden on top and bubbling when cooked. Serve warm with sour cream and sliced avocado.

Nutrition: Calories: 416; Protein: 32g; Fiber: 3g; Fat: 22g; Carbs: 5g

Lime Chicken Thighs

Preparation Time: 37 minutes
Servings: 4
Ingredients:

4 bone-in, skin-on chicken thighs
2 medium limes
¼ cup chopped fresh cilantro
2 tsp. chili powder
1 tsp. cumin
1 tsp. baking powder.
½ tsp. garlic powder.

Directions:

Pat chicken thighs dry and sprinkle with baking powder.

In a small bowl, mix garlic powder, chili powder and cumin and sprinkle evenly over thighs, gently rubbing on and under chicken skin

Cut one lime in half and squeeze juice over thighs. Place chicken into the air fryer basket.
Adjust the temperature to 380 Degrees F and set the timer for 22 minutes

Cut other lime into four wedges for serving and garnish cooked chicken with wedges and cilantro.
Nutrition: Calories: 435; Protein: 33g; Fiber: 6g; Fat: 21g; Carbs: 6g

Cajun Chicken Tenders

Preparation Time: 27 minutes
Servings: 4
Ingredients:
1 lb. boneless, skinless chicken tenders
¼ cup full-fat ranch dressing
2 tbsp. coconut oil
⅛ tsp. ground cayenne pepper
½ tsp. dried thyme
¼ tsp. onion powder.
½ tsp. garlic powder.
2 tsp. paprika
1 tsp. chili powder
Directions:
In a small bowl, combine all seasonings.
Drizzle oil over chicken tenders and then generously coat each tender in the spice mixture. Place tenders into the air fryer basket
Adjust the temperature to 375 Degrees F and set the timer for 17 minutes
Tenders will be 165 Degrees F internally when fully cooked.
Serve with ranch dressing for dipping.
Nutrition: Calories: 163; Protein: 22g; Fiber: 8g; Fat: 5g; Carbs: 5g

Thyme Duck Legs

Preparation Time: 35 minutes
Servings: 4
Ingredients:
4 duck legs
2 tbsp. olive oil
4 tsp. thyme; dried
3 tsp. fennel seeds, crushed
A pinch of salt and black pepper
Directions:
Take a bowl and mix the duck legs with all the other **Ingredients:** and toss well.
Put the duck legs in your air fryer's basket and cook at 380°F for 15 minutes on each side. Divide between plates and serve
Nutrition: Calories: 274; Fat: 11g; Fiber: 4g; Carbs: 6g; Protein: 14g

Chicken Cordon Bleu Casserole

Preparation Time: 30 minutes
Servings: 4
Ingredients:
2 cups cubed cooked chicken thigh meat
2 oz. Swiss cheese, cubed
1 oz. pork rinds, crushed
4 oz. full-fat cream cheese; softened.
½ cup cubed cooked ham
2 tbsp. unsalted butter; melted.
1 tbsp. heavy cream

2 tsp. Dijon mustard

Directions:

Place chicken and ham into a 6-inch round baking pan and toss so meat is evenly mixed. Sprinkle cheese cubes on top of meat

Take a large bowl, mix cream cheese, heavy cream, butter and mustard and then pour the mixture over the meat and cheese. Top with pork rinds. Place pan into the air fryer basket. Adjust the temperature to 350 Degrees F and set the timer for 15 minutes

The casserole will be browned and bubbling when done. Serve warm.

Nutrition: Calories: 403; Protein: 37g; Fiber: 0g; Fat: 22g; Carbs: 3g

Spicy Chicken Tenders with Aioli Sauce

Preparation Time: 15 minutes

Servings: 4

Ingredients:

3 chicken breasts, skinless, cut into strips

4 tbsp olive oil

1 cup breadcrumbs

Salt and black pepper to taste

½ tbsp garlic powder

½ tbsp ground chili

Prep + Cook Time½ cup mayonnaise

2 tbsp olive oil

½ tbsp ground chili

Directions:

Mix breadcrumbs, salt, pepper, garlic powder and chili, and spread onto a plate. Spray the chicken with oil. Roll the strips in the breadcrumb mixture until well coated. Spray with a little bit of oil.

Arrange an even layer of strips into your air fryer and cook for 6 minutes at 360 F, turning once halfway through. To prepare the hot aioli: combine mayo with oil and ground chili. Serve hot.

Marinara Sauce Cheese Chicken

Preparation Time: 25 minutes

Servings: 2

Ingredients:

2 chicken breasts, skinless, beaten, ½-inch thick

1 egg, beaten

½ cup breadcrumbs

A pinch of salt and black pepper

2 tbsp marinara sauce

2 tbsp Grana Padano cheese, grated

2 slices mozzarella cheese

Directions:

Dip the breasts into the egg, then into the crumbs and arrange in the fryer; cook for 5 minutes at 400 F. Then, turn over and drizzle with marinara sauce, Grana Padano and mozzarella. Cook for 5 more minutes at 400 F.

Honey Thighs with Garlic

Preparation Time: 30 minutes
Servings: 4
Ingredients:
4 thighs, skin-on
3 tbsp honey
2 tbsp Dijon mustard
½ tbsp garlic powder
Salt and black pepper to taste
Directions:
In a bowl, mix honey, mustard, garlic, salt, and black pepper. Coat the thighs in the mixture and arrange them in your air fryer. Cook for 16 minutes at 400 F, turning once halfway through.

Buttery Chicken with Monterrey Jack Cheese

Preparation Time: 30 minutes
Servings: 4
Ingredients:
½ cup Italian breadcrumbs
2 tbsp grated Parmesan cheese
1 tbsp butter, melted
4 chicken thighs
½ cup marinara sauce
½ cup shredded Monterrey Jack cheese
Directions:
Spray the air fryer basket with cooking spray. In a bowl, mix the crumbs and Parmesan cheese. Pour the butter into another bowl. Brush the thighs with butter. Dip each one into the crumbs mixture, until well-coated.
Arrange two chicken thighs in the air fryer, and lightly spray with cooking oil. Cook for 5 minutes at 380 F. Flip over, top with a few tbsp marinara sauce and shredded Monterrey Jack cheese. Cook until no longer pink in the center, for 4 minutes. Repeat with the remaining thighs.

Chicken Breasts with Rosemary

Preparation Time: 30minutes
Servings: 2
Ingredients:
2 tbsp Dijon mustard
1 tbsp maple syrup
2 tsp minced fresh rosemary
¼ tsp salt
⅛ tsp black pepper
2 chicken breasts, boneless, skinless
Directions:
In a bowl, mix mustard, maple syrup, rosemary, salt, and pepper. Rub mixture onto chicken breasts. Spray generously the air fryer basket generously with cooking spray. Arrange the breasts inside and cook for 20 minutes, turning once halfway through.

Thyme Whole Chicken with Pancetta and Lemon

Preparation Time: 60 minutes
Servings: 4
Ingredients:
1 small whole chicken
1 lemon
4 slices pancetta, roughly chopped
1 onion, chopped
1 sprig fresh thyme
Olive oil
Salt and black pepper
Directions:
In a bowl, mix pancetta, onion, thyme, salt, and black pepper. Pat dry the chicken with a dry paper towel. Insert the pancetta mixture into chicken's cavity and press tight.
Put in the whole lemon, and rub the top and sides of the chicken with salt and black pepper. Spray the air fryer's basket with olive oil and arrange the chicken inside. Cook for 30 minutes on 400 F, turning once halfway through.

Green Chicken Drumsticks with Coconut Cream

Preparation Time: 25 minutes
Servings: 4
Ingredients:
4 chicken drumsticks, boneless, skinless
2 tbsp green curry paste
3 tbsp coconut cream
Salt and black pepper
½ fresh jalapeno chili, finely chopped
A handful of fresh parsley, roughly chopped
Directions:
In a bowl, add drumsticks, paste, cream, salt, black pepper and jalapeno; coat the chicken well. Arrange the drumsticks in the air fryer and cook for 6 minutes at 400 F, flipping once halfway through. Serve with fresh cilantro.

Creamy Chicken Nuggets

Preparation Time: 15 minutes
Servings: 4
Ingredients:
2 chicken breasts, skinless, boneless, cut into nuggets
4 tbsp sour cream
½ cup breadcrumbs
½ tbsp garlic powder
½ tsp cayenne pepper
Salt and black pepper to taste
Directions:
In a bowl, add sour cream and place the chicken. Stir well. Mix the breadcrumbs, garlic, cayenne, salt, and black pepper and scatter onto a plate. Roll up the chicken in the breadcrumbs to coat well. Grease the air with oil. Arrange the nuggets in an even layer and cook for 10 minutes on 360 F, turning once halfway through cooking.

Herby Stuffed Chicken

Preparation Time: 50 minutes
Servings: 2
Ingredients:
1 small chicken
1 ½ tbsp olive oil
Salt and black pepper to taste to season
1 cup breadcrumbs
⅓ cup chopped sage
⅓ cup chopped thyme
2 cloves garlic, crushed
1 brown onion, chopped
3 tbsp butter
2 eggs, beaten
Directions:
Rinse the chicken gently, pat dry with a paper towel and remove any excess fat with a knife; set aside. On a stove top, place a pan. Add the butter, garlic and onion and sauté to brown. Add the eggs, sage, thyme, pepper, and salt.
Mix well. Cook for 20 seconds and turn the heat off. Stuff the chicken with the mixture into the cavity. Then, tie the legs of the spatchcock with a butcher's twine and brush with olive oil. Rub the top and sides of the chicken generously with salt and pepper. Preheat the Air Fryer to 390 F. Place the spatchcock into the fryer basket and roast for 25 minutes. Turn the chicken over and continue cooking for 10-15 minutes more; check throughout the cooking time to ensure it doesn't dry or overcooks. Remove onto a chopping board and wrap it with aluminum foil; let rest for 10 minutes. Serve with a side of steamed broccoli.

Chili Chicken Wings

Preparation Time: 16 hrs 40 minutes
Servings: 4
Ingredients:
2 lb chicken wings
1 tbsp olive oil
3 cloves garlic, minced
1 tbsp chili powder
½ tbsp cinnamon powder
½ tsp allspice
1 habanero pepper, seeded
1 tbsp soy sauce
½ tbsp white pepper
¼ cup red wine vinegar
3 tbsp lime juice
2 Scallions, chopped
½ tbsp grated ginger
½ tbsp chopped fresh thyme
⅓ tbsp sugar
½ tbsp salt
Directions:
In a bowl, add the olive oil, soy sauce, garlic, habanero pepper, allspice, cinnamon powder, cayenne pepper, white pepper, salt, sugar, thyme, ginger, scallions, lime juice, and red wine vinegar; mix well.

Add the chicken wings to the marinade mixture and coat it well with the mixture. Cover the bowl with cling film and refrigerate the chicken to marinate for 16 hours. Preheat the Air Fryer to 400 F. Remove the chicken from the fridge, drain all the liquid, and pat each wing dry using a paper towel.

Place half of the wings in the basket and cook for 16 minutes. Shake halfway through. Remove onto a serving platter and repeat the cooking process for the remaining wings. Serve with blue cheese dip or ranch dressing.

Spice and Juicy Chicken Breasts

Preparation Time: 35 minutes
Servings: 3
Ingredients:

2 chicken breasts
Salt and black pepper to taste
1 cup flour
3 eggs
½ cup apple cider vinegar
½ tbsp ginger paste
½ tbsp garlic paste
1 tbsp sugar
2 red chilies, minced
2 tbsp tomato puree
1 red pepper
1 green pepper
1 tbsp paprika
4 tbsp water

Directions:

Preheat the Air Fryer to 350 F. Put the chicken breasts on a clean flat surface. Cut them in cubes. Pour the flour in a bowl, crack the eggs in, add the salt and pepper; whisk. Put the chicken in the flour mixture; mix to coat.

Place the chicken in the fryer's basket, spray with cooking spray, and fry for 8 minutes. Pull out the fryer basket, shake to toss, and spray again with cooking spray. Keep cooking for 7 minutes or until golden and crispy.

Remove the chicken to a plate. Put the red, yellow, and green peppers on a chopping board. Using a knife, cut open and deseed them; cut the flesh in long strips. In a bowl, add the water, apple cider vinegar, sugar, ginger and garlic puree, red chili, tomato puree, and smoked paprika; mix with a fork.

Place a skillet over medium heat on a stovetop and spray with cooking spray. Add the chicken and pepper strips. Stir and cook until the peppers are sweaty but still crunchy. Pour the chili mixture on the chicken, stir, and bring to simmer for 10 minutes; turn off the heat. Dish the chicken chili sauce into a serving bowl and serve.

Chicken Kabobs with Garlic Sauce

Preparation Time: 35 minutes
Servings: 3
Ingredients:

3 chicken breasts
Salt to season
1 tbsp chili powder
¼ cup maple syrup
½ cup soy sauce

2 red peppers
1 green pepper
7 mushrooms
2 tbsp sesame seeds
Prep + Cook Time1 garlic clove
2 tbsp olive oil
Zest and juice from 1 lime
A pinch of salt
¼ cup fresh parsley, chopped

Directions:

Put the chicken breasts on a clean flat surface and cut them in 2-inch cubes with a knife. Add them to a bowl, along with the chili powder, salt, maple syrup, soy sauce, sesame seeds, and spray them with cooking spray. Toss to coat and set aside. Place the peppers on the chopping board. Use a knife to open, deseed and cut in cubes.

Likewise, cut the mushrooms in halves. Start stacking up the **Ingredients:** - stick 1 red pepper, then green, a chicken cube, and a mushroom half. Repeat the arrangement until the skewer is full. Repeat the process until all the **Ingredients:** are used. Preheat the Air Fryer to 330 F.

Brush the kabobs with soy sauce mixture and place them into the fryer basket. Grease with cooking spray and grill for 20 minutes; flip halfway through. Meanwhile, mix all salsa verde **Ingredients:** in your food processor and blend until you obtain a chunky paste. Remove the kabobs when ready and serve with a side of salsa verde.

Zucchini Stuffed Lemony Chicken

Preparation Time: 100 minutes
Servings: 6
Ingredients:

Prep + Cook Time1 whole chicken, 3 lb
2 red and peeled onions
2 tbsp olive oil
2 apricots
1 zucchini
1 apple
2 cloves finely chopped garlic
Fresh chopped thyme
Salt and black pepper to taste
Prep + Cook TimePrep + Cook Time5 oz honey
juice from 1 lemon
2 tbsp olive oil
Salt and black pepper to taste

Directions:

For the stuffing, chop all **Ingredients:** into tiny pieces. Transfer to a large bowl and add the olive oil. Season with salt and black pepper. Fill the cavity of the chicken with the stuffing, without packing it tightly.

Place the chicken in the Air Fryer and cook for 35 minutes at 340 F. Warm the honey and the lemon juice in a large pan; season with salt and pepper. Reduce the temperature of the Air Fryer to 320 F.

Brush the chicken with some of the honey-lemon marinade and return it to the fryer. Cook for another 70 minutes; brush the chicken every 20-25 minutes with the marinade. Garnish with parsley, and serve with potatoes.

Drumsticks with Blue Cheese Sauce

Preparation Time: 2 hrs 25 minutes
Servings: 4
Ingredients:
Prep + Cook Time1 lb mini drumsticks
3 tbsp butter
3 tbsp paprika
2 tbsp powdered cumin
¼ cup hot sauce
1 tbsp maple syrup
2 tbsp onion powder
2 tbsp garlic powder
Prep + Cook Time½ cup mayonnaise
1 cup crumbled blue cheese
1 cup sour cream
1 ½ tbsp garlic powder
1 ½ tbsp onion powder
Salt and black pepper to taste
1 ½ tbsp cayenne pepper
1 ½ tbsp white wine vinegar
2 tbsp buttermilk
1 ½ worcestershire sauce
Directions:
Start with the drumstick sauce; place a pan over medium heat on a stove top. Melt the butter, and add the hot sauce, paprika, garlic, onion, maple syrup, and cumin; mix well. Cook the mixture for 5 minutes or until the sauce reduces. Turn off the heat and let cool. Put the drumsticks in a bowl, pour half of the sauce over, and mix it.
Save the remaining sauce for serving. Refrigerate the drumsticks for 2 hours. Meanwhile, make the blue cheese sauce: in a jug, add the sour cream, blue cheese, mayonnaise, garlic powder, onion powder, buttermilk, cayenne pepper, vinegar, Worcestershire sauce, pepper, and salt. Using a stick blender, blend the **Ingredients:** until they are well mixed with no large lumps. Adjust the salt and pepper taste as desired. Preheat the Air Fryer to 350 F.
Remove the drumsticks from the fridge and place them in the fryer basket; cook for 15 minutes. Turn the drumsticks with tongs every 5 minutes to ensure that they are evenly cooked. Remove the drumsticks to a serving bowl and pour the remaining sauce over. Serve with the blue cheese sauce and a side of celery sticks.

Chili Lime Chicken Lollipop

Preparation Time: 50 minutes
Servings: 3
Ingredients:
1 lb mini chicken drumsticks
½ tbsp soy sauce
1 tbsp lime juice
Salt and black pepper to taste
1 tbsp cornstarch
½ tbsp minced garlic
½ tbsp chili powder
½ tbsp chopped cilantro
½ tbsp garlic- ginger paste

1 tbsp vinegar
1 tbsp chili paste
½ tbsp beaten egg
1 tbsp paprika
1 tbsp flour
2 tbsp maple syrup

Directions:

Mix garlic ginger paste, chili powder, maple syrup, paprika powder, chopped coriander, plain vinegar, egg, garlic, and salt, in a bowl. Add the chicken drumsticks and toss to coat; Stir in cornstarch, flour, and lime juice.

Preheat the Air Fryer to 350 F. Remove each drumstick, shake off the excess marinade, and place in a single layer in the basket; cook for 5 minutes. Slide out the basket, spray the chicken with cooking spray and continue to cook for 5 minutes. Remove onto a serving platter and serve with tomato dip and a side of steamed asparagus.

Almond Turkey with Lemon and Eggs

Preparation Time: 50 minutes
Servings: 3
Ingredients:

1 lb turkey breasts
Salt and black pepper to taste to season
¼ cup chicken soup cream
¼ cup mayonnaise
2 tbsp lemon juice
¼ cup slivered almonds, chopped
¼ cup breadcrumbs
2 tbsp chopped green onion
2 tbsp chopped pimentos
2 Boiled eggs, chopped
½ cup diced celery

Directions:

Preheat the Air Fryer to 390 F. Place the turkey breasts on a clean flat surface and season with salt and pepper.

Grease with cooking spray and place them in the fryer's basket; cook for 13 minutes. Remove turkey back onto the chopping board, let cool, and cut into dices. In a bowl, add the celery, chopped eggs, pimentos, green onions, slivered almonds, lemon juice, mayonnaise, diced turkey, and chicken soup cream and mix well.

Grease a 5 X 5 inches casserole dish with cooking spray, scoop the turkey mixture into the bowl, sprinkle the breadcrumbs on it, and spray with cooking spray. Put the dish in the fryer basket, and bake the **Ingredients:** at 390 F for 20 minutes. Remove and serve with a side of steamed asparagus.

Party Chicken Wings with Sesame

Preparation Time: 25 minutes
Servings: 4
Ingredients:

1 lb chicken wings
2 tbsp sesame oil
2 tbsp maple syrup
Salt and black pepper
3 tbsp sesame seeds

Directions:
In a bowl, add wings, oil, maple syrup, salt and pepper, and stir to coat well. In another bowl, add the sesame seeds and roll the wings in the seeds to coat thoroughly. Arrange the wings in an even layer inside your air fryer and cook for 12 minutes on 360 F, turning once halfway through.

Buttermilk Chicken Bites

Preparation Time: 25 minutes
Servings: 4
Ingredients:
2 chicken breasts, skinless, cut into 2 pieces each
1 egg, beaten
¼ cup buttermilk
1 cup corn flakes, crushed
Salt and black pepper to taste
Directions:
In a bowl, whisk egg and buttermilk. Add in chicken pieces and stir to coat. In a plate, spread the cornflakes out and mix with salt and pepper. Coat the chicken pieces in the cornflakes. Spray the air fryer with cooking spray.
Arrange the chicken in an even layer in the air fryer; cook for 12 minutes at 360 F, turning once halfway through.

Savory Chicken Burgers

Preparation Time: 25 minutes
Servings: 4
Ingredients:
1 lb ground chicken
½ onion, chopped
2 garlic cloves, chopped
1 egg, beaten
½ cup breadcrumbs
½ tbsp ground cumin
½ tbsp paprika
½ tbsp cilantro seeds, crushed
Salt and black pepper to taste
Directions:
In a bowl, mix chicken, onion, garlic, egg, breadcrumbs, cumin, paprika, cilantro, salt, and black pepper, with hands; shape into 4 patties. Grease the air fryer with oil, and arrange the patties inside. Do not layer them. Cook in batches if needed. Cook for 10 minutes at 380 F, turning once halfway through.

Creamy Chicken With Prosciutto

Preparation Time: 25 minutes
Servings: 2
Ingredients:
2 chicken breasts
1 tbsp olive oil
Salt and black pepper to taste to season
1 cup semi-dried tomatoes, sliced
½ cup brie cheese, halved
4 slices thin prosciutto

Directions:

Preheat the Air Fryer to 365 F. Put the chicken on a chopping board, and cut a small incision deep enough to make stuffing on both. Insert one slice of cheese and 4 to 5 tomato slices into each chicken.

Lay the prosciutto on the chopping board. Put the chicken on one side and roll the prosciutto over the chicken making sure that both ends of the prosciutto meet under the chicken.

Drizzle olive oil and sprinkle with salt and pepper. Place the chicken in the basket and cook for 10 minutes. Turn the breasts over and cook for another 5 minutes. Slice each chicken breast in half and serve with tomato salad.

Chicken Tenders with Tarragon

Preparation Time: 15minutes

Servings: 2

Ingredients:

2 chicken tenders

Salt and black pepper to taste

½ cup dried tarragon

1 tbsp butter

Directions:

Preheat the Air Fryer to 390 F. Lay out a 12 X 12 inch cut of foil on a flat surface. Place the chicken breasts on the foil, sprinkle the tarragon on both, and share the butter onto both breasts. Sprinkle with salt and pepper.

Loosely wrap the foil around the breasts to enable air flow. Place the wrapped chicken in the basket and cook for 12 minutes. Remove the chicken and carefully unwrap the foil. Serve with the sauce extract and steamed veggies.

Herby Chicken with Lime

Preparation Time: 50 minutes

Servings: 4

Ingredients:

1 (2½ lbwhole chicken, on the bone

Salt and black pepper to taste to season

1 tbsp chili powder

1 tbsp garlic powder

4 tbsp oregano

2 tbsp cilantro powder

2 tbsp cumin powder

2 tbsp olive oil

4 tbsp paprika

1 lime, juiced

Directions:

In a bowl, pour the oregano, garlic powder, chili powder, ground cilantro, paprika, cumin powder, pepper, salt, and olive oil. Mix well to create a rub for the chicken, and rub onto it. Refrigerate for 20 minutes.

Preheat the Air Fryer to 350 F. Remove the chicken from the refrigerator; place in the fryer basket and cook for 20 minutes. Use a skewer to poke the chicken to ensure that it is clear of juices. If not, cook the chicken further for 5 to 10 minutes; let to rest for 10 minutes. After, drizzle the lime juice over and serve with green salad.

Chicken Wrapped In Bacon

Preparation Time: 20 minutes
Servings: 2 to 4
Ingredients:
2 chicken breasts
8 oz onion and chive cream cheese
1 tbsp butter
6 turkey bacon
Salt to taste
1 tbsp fresh parsley, chopped
juice from ½ lemon
Directions:
Preheat the Air Fryer to 390 F. Stretch out the bacon slightly and lay them on in 2 sets; 3 bacon strips together on each side. Place the chicken breast on each bacon set and use a knife to smear the cream cheese on both. Share the butter on top and sprinkle with salt. Wrap the bacon around the chicken and secure the ends into the wrap.
Place the wrapped chicken in the fryer's basket and cook for 14 minutes. Turn the chicken halfway through. Remove the chicken onto a serving platter and top with parsley and lemon juice. Serve with steamed greens.

Fruity Chicken Breasts with BBQ Sauce

Preparation Time: 20 minutes
Servings: 2
Ingredients:
2 large chicken breasts, cubed
2 green bell peppers, sliced
½ onion, sliced
1 can drain pineapple chunks
½ cup barbecue sauce
Directions:
Preheat the Air Fryer to 370 F. Thread the green bell peppers, the chicken, the onions and the pineapple chunks on the skewers. Brush with barbecue sauce and fry for 20 minutes, until thoroughly cooked and slightly crispy.

Broccoli Chicken Casserole

Preparation Time: 45 minutes
Servings: 3
Ingredients:
3 chicken breasts
Salt and black pepper to taste
1 cup shredded Cheddar cheese
1 broccoli head
½ cup mushroom soup cream
½ cup croutons
Directions:
Preheat the Air Fryer to 390 F. Place the chicken breasts on a clean flat surface and season with salt and pepper. Grease with cooking spray and place them in the fryer basket. Close the Air Fryer and cook for 13 minutes. Meanwhile, place the broccoli on the chopping board and use a knife to chop.

Remove them onto the chopping board, let cool, and cut into bite-size pieces. In a bowl, add the chicken, broccoli, cheddar cheese, and mushroom soup cream; mix well. Scoop the mixture into a 3 X 3cm casserole dish, add the croutons on top and spray with cooking spray. Put the dish in the basket and cook for 10 minutes. Serve with a side of steamed greens.

5Asian Spicy Turkey

Preparation Time: 35 minutes
Servings: 6
Nutrition: 279 Calories; 12g Fat; 4g Carbs; 29g Protein; 4g Sugars; 2g Fiber
Ingredients:
1 tablespoon sesame oil
2 pounds turkey thighs
1 teaspoon Chinese Five-spice powder
1 teaspoon pink Himalayan salt
1/4 teaspoon Sichuan pepper
1 tablespoon Chinese rice vinegar
2 tablespoons soy sauce
1 tablespoon chili sauce
1 tablespoon mustard
Directions:
Preheat your Air Fryer to 360 degrees F.
Brush the sesame oil all over the turkey thighs. Season them with spices.
Cook for 23 minutes, turning over once or twice. Make sure to work in batches to ensure even cooking
In the meantime, combine the remaining **Ingredients:** in a wok (or similar type panthat is preheated over medium-high heat. Cook and stir until the sauce reduces by about a third.
Add the fried turkey thighs to the wok; gently stir to coat with the sauce.
Let the turkey rest for 10 minutes before slicing and serving. Enjoy!

5Spicy Chicken Drumsticks with Herbs

Preparation Time: 40 minutes
Servings: 6
Nutrition: 280 Calories; 17g Fat; 6g Carbs; 21g Protein; 4g Sugars; 5g Fiber
Ingredients:
6 chicken drumsticks
Sauce:
6 ounces hot sauce
3 tablespoons olive oil
3 tablespoons tamari sauce
1 teaspoon dried thyme
1/2 teaspoon dried oregano
Directions:
Spritz the sides and bottom of the cooking basket with a nonstick cooking spray.
Cook the chicken drumsticks at 380 degrees F for 35 minutes, flipping them over halfway through.
Meanwhile, heat the hot sauce, olive oil, tamari sauce, thyme, and oregano in a pan over medium-low heat; reserve.
Drizzle the sauce over the prepared chicken drumsticks; toss to coat well and serve. Bon appétit!

5Classic Chicken with Peanuts

Preparation Time: 25 minutes
Servings: 4
Nutrition: 354 Calories; 14g Fat; 3g Carbs; 40g Protein; 4g Sugars; 7g Fiber
Ingredients:
1 ½ pounds chicken tenderloins
2 tablespoons peanut oil
1/2 cup parmesan cheese, grated
Sea salt and ground black pepper, to taste
1/2 teaspoon garlic powder
1 teaspoon red pepper flakes
2 tablespoons peanuts, roasted and roughly chopped
Directions:
Start by preheating your Air Fryer to 360 degrees F.
Brush the chicken tenderloins with peanut oil on all sides.
In a mixing bowl, thoroughly combine grated parmesan cheese, salt, black pepper, garlic powder, and red pepper flakes. Dredge the chicken in the breading, shaking off any residual coating.
Lay the chicken tenderloins into the cooking basket. Cook for 12 to 13 minutes or until it is no longer pink in the center. Work in batches; an instant-read thermometer should read at least 165 degrees F.
Serve garnished with roasted peanuts. Bon appétit!

5Turkey with Paprika and Tarragon

Preparation Time: 40 minutes
Servings: 6
Nutrition: 217 Calories; 5g Fat; 2g Carbs; 37g Protein; 5g Sugars; 3g Fiber
Ingredients:
2 pounds turkey tenderloins
2 tablespoons olive oil
Salt and ground black pepper, to taste
1 teaspoon smoked paprika
2 tablespoons dry white wine
1 tablespoon fresh tarragon leaves, chopped
Directions:
Brush the turkey tenderloins with olive oil. Season with salt, black pepper, and paprika.
Afterwards, add the white wine and tarragon.
Cook the turkey tenderloins at 350 degrees F for 30 minutes, flipping them over halfway through.
Let them rest for 5 to 9 minutes before slicing and serving. Enjoy!

5Italian-Style Chicken with Roma Tomatoes

Preparation Time: 45 minutes
Servings: 8
Nutrition: 315 Calories; 11g Fat; 7g Carbs; 36g Protein; 7g Sugars; 9g Fiber
Ingredients:
2 teaspoons olive oil, melted
3 pounds chicken breasts, bone-in
1/2 teaspoon black pepper, freshly ground
1/2 teaspoon salt

1 teaspoon cayenne pepper
2 tablespoons fresh parsley, minced
1 teaspoon fresh basil, minced
1 teaspoon fresh rosemary, minced
4 medium-sized Roma tomatoes, halved

Directions:

Start by preheating your Air Fryer to 370 degrees F. Brush the cooking basket with 1 teaspoon of olive oil.

Sprinkle the chicken breasts with all seasonings listed above.

Cook for 25 minutes or until chicken breasts are slightly browned. Work in batches.

Arrange the tomatoes in the cooking basket and brush them with the remaining teaspoon of olive oil. Season with sea salt.

Cook the tomatoes at 350 degrees F for 10 minutes, shaking halfway through the cooking time. Serve with chicken breasts. Bon appétit!

5Duck Breasts with Candy Onion and Coriander

Preparation Time: 25 minutes
Servings: 4
Nutrition: 362 Calories; 17g Fat; 4g Carbs; 43g Protein; 3g Sugars; 5g Fiber

Ingredients:

1 ½ pounds duck breasts, skin removed
1 teaspoon kosher salt
1/2 teaspoon cayenne pepper
1/3 teaspoon black pepper
1/2 teaspoon smoked paprika
1 tablespoon Thai red curry paste
1 cup candy onions, halved
1/4 small pack coriander, chopped

Directions:

Place the duck breasts between 2 sheets of foil; then, use a rolling pin to bash the duck until they are 1-inch thick.

Preheat your Air Fryer to 395 degrees F.

Rub the duck breasts with salt, cayenne pepper, black pepper, paprika, and red curry paste. Place the duck breast in the cooking basket.

Cook for 11 to 12 minutes. Top with candy onions and cook for another 10 to 11 minutes.

Serve garnished with coriander and enjoy!

6Paprika Chicken Legs with Turnip

Preparation Time: 30 minutes
Servings: 3

Nutrition: 207 Calories; 8g Fat; 4g Carbs; 25g Protein; 6g Sugars; 5g Fiber

Ingredients:

1 pound chicken legs
1 teaspoon Himalayan salt
1 teaspoon paprika
1/2 teaspoon ground black pepper
1 teaspoon butter, melted
1 turnip, trimmed and sliced

Directions:

Spritz the sides and bottom of the cooking basket with a nonstick cooking spray.

Season the chicken legs with salt, paprika, and ground black pepper.

Cook at 370 degrees F for 10 minutes. Increase the temperature to 380 degrees F.

Drizzle turnip slices with melted butter and transfer them to the cooking basket with the chicken.

Cook the turnips and chicken for 15 minutes more, flipping them halfway through the cooking time.

As for the chicken, an instant-read thermometer should read at least 165 degrees F.

Serve and enjoy!

6Turkey Burgers with Crispy Bacon

Preparation Time: 30 minutes

Servings: 4

Nutrition: 308 Calories; 14g Fat; 4g Carbs; 39g Protein; 4g Sugars; 6g Fiber

Ingredients:

2 tablespoons vermouth

2 strips Canadian bacon, sliced

1 pound ground turkey

1/2 shallot, minced

2 garlic cloves, minced

2 tablespoons fish sauce

Sea salt and ground black pepper, to taste

1 teaspoon red pepper flakes

4 tablespoons tomato ketchup

4 tablespoons mayonnaise

4 (1-ounceslices Cheddar cheese

4 lettuce leaves

Directions:

Start by preheating your Air Fryer to 400 degrees F. Brush the Canadian bacon with the vermouth.

Cook for 3 minutes. Flip the bacon over and cook an additional 3 minutes.

Then, thoroughly combine the ground turkey, shallots, garlic, fish sauce, salt, black pepper, and red pepper. Form the meat mixture into 4 burger patties.

Bake in the preheated Air Fryer at 370 degrees F for 10 minutes. Flip them over and cook another 10 minutes.

Serve turkey burgers with the ketchup, mayonnaise, bacon, cheese and lettuce; serve immediately.

6Chicken Sausage Casserole

Preparation Time: 50 minutes

Servings: 4

Nutrition: 300 Calories; 18g Fat; 7g Carbs; 23g Protein; 7g Sugars; 3g Fiber

Ingredients:

8 ounces zucchini, spiralized

1 pound smoked chicken sausage, sliced

1 tomato, pureed

1/2 cup Asiago cheese, shredded

1 tablespoon Italian seasoning mix

3 tablespoons Romano cheese, grated

1 tablespoon fresh basil leaves, chiffonade

Directions:
Salt the zucchini and let it stand for 30 minutes; pat it dry with kitchen towels.
Then, spritz a baking pan with cooking spray; add the zucchini to the pan. Stir in the chicken sausage, tomato puree, Asiago cheese, and Italian seasoning mix.
Bake in the preheated Air Fryer at 325 degrees F for 11 minutes.
Top with the grated Romano cheese. Turn the temperature to 390 degrees F and cook an additional 5 minutes or until everything is thoroughly heated and the cheese is melted.
Garnish with fresh basil leaves. Bon appétit!

6Turkey Tenderloins with Gravy

Preparation Time: 50 minutes
Servings: 4
Nutrition: 276 Calories; 16,4g Fat; 2g Carbs; 29g Protein; 3g Sugars; 9g Fiber
Ingredients:
1 pound turkey tenderloins
1 tablespoon Dijon-style mustard
1 tablespoon olive oil
Sea salt and ground black pepper, to taste
1 teaspoon Italian seasoning mix
1 cup turkey stock
1/2 teaspoon xanthan gum
4 tablespoons tomato ketchup
4 tablespoons mayonnaise
4 pickles, sliced
Directions:
Rub the turkey tenderloins with the mustard and olive oil. Season with salt, black pepper, and Italian seasoning mix.
Cook the turkey tenderloins at 350 degrees F for 30 minutes, flipping them over halfway through. Let them rest for 5 to 7 minutes before slicing.
For the gravy, in a saucepan, place the drippings from the roasted turkey. Add in turkey stock and bring to a boil.
Stir in xanthan gum and whisk to combine. Let simmer another 5 to 10 minutes until starting to thicken. Gravy will thicken more as it cools.
Serve turkey tenderloins with gravy, tomato ketchup, mayonnaise, and pickles. Serve and enjoy!

6Old-Fashioned Turkey Chili

Preparation Time: 40 minutes
Servings: 4
Nutrition: 271 Calories; 17g Fat; 6g Carbs; 27g Protein; 6g Sugars; 4g Fiber
Ingredients:
1/2 medium-sized leek, chopped
1/2 red onion, chopped
2 garlic cloves, minced
1 jalapeno pepper, seeded and minced
1 bell pepper, seeded and chopped
2 tablespoons olive oil
1 pound ground turkey, 85% lean 15% fat
2 cups tomato puree
2 cups chicken stock
1/2 teaspoon black peppercorns

Salt, to taste
1 teaspoon chili powder
1 teaspoon mustard seeds
1 teaspoon ground cumin
Directions:
Start by preheating your Air Fryer to 365 degrees F.
Place the leeks, onion, garlic and peppers in a baking pan; drizzle olive oil evenly over the top. Cook for 4 to 6 minutes.
Add the ground turkey. Cook for 6 minutes more or until the meat is no longer pink.
Now, add the tomato puree, 1 cup of chicken stock, black peppercorns, salt, chili powder, mustard seeds, and cumin to the baking pan. Cook for 24 minutes, stirring every 7 to 10 minutes.
Bon appétit!

6Rustic Chicken Drumettes with Chives

Preparation Time: 30 minutes
Servings: 3
Nutrition: 319 Calories; 13g Fat; 4g Carbs; 45g Protein; 5g Sugars; 4g Fiber
Ingredients:
1/3 cup almond meal
1/2 teaspoon ground white pepper
1 teaspoon seasoning salt
1 teaspoon garlic paste
1 teaspoon rosemary
1 whole egg + 1 egg white
6 chicken drumettes
1 heaping tablespoon fresh chives, chopped
Directions:
Start by preheating your Air Fryer to 390 degrees.
Mix the almond meal with white pepper, salt, garlic paste, and rosemary in a small-sized bowl.
In another bowl, beat the eggs until frothy.
Dip the chicken into the flour mixture, then into the beaten eggs; coat with the flour mixture one more time.
Cook the chicken drumettes for 22 minutes. Serve warm, garnished with chives.

6Piri Piri Chicken

Preparation Time: 1 hour 30 minutes
Servings: 6
Nutrition: 517 Calories; 21g Fat; 9g Carbs; 47g Protein; 6g Sugars; 4g Fiber
Ingredients:
12 chicken wings
1 ½ ounces butter, melted
1 teaspoon onion powder
1/2 teaspoon cumin powder
1 teaspoon garlic paste
For the Sauce:
2 ounces piri piri peppers, stemmed and chopped
1 tablespoon pimiento, deveined and minced
1 garlic clove, chopped
2 tablespoons fresh lemon juice
1/3 teaspoon sea salt

1/2 teaspoon tarragon

Directions:

Steam the chicken wings using a steamer basket that is placed over a saucepan with boiling water; reduce the heat.

Now, steam the wings for 10 minutes over a moderate heat. Toss the wings with butter, onion powder, cumin powder, and garlic paste.

Let the chicken wings cool to room temperature. Then, refrigerate them for 45 to 50 minutes.

Roast in the preheated Air Fryer at 330 degrees F for 25 to 30 minutes; make sure to flip them halfway through.

While the chicken wings are cooking, prepare the sauce by mixing all of the sauce **Ingredients:** in a food processor. Toss the wings with prepared Piri Piri Sauce and serve.

6Chicken Sausage in Dijon Sauce

Preparation Time: 20 minutes

Servings: 4

Nutrition: 575 Calories; 52g Fat; 5g Carbs; 24g Protein; 8g Sugars; 5g Fiber

Ingredients:

4 chicken sausages

1/4 cup mayonnaise

2 tablespoons Dijon mustard

1 tablespoon balsamic vinegar

1/2 teaspoon dried rosemary

Directions:

Arrange the sausages on the grill pan and transfer it to the preheated Air Fryer.

Grill the sausages at 350 degrees F for approximately 13 minutes. Turn them halfway through cooking.

Meanwhile, prepare the sauce by mixing the remaining **Ingredients:** with a wire whisk. Serve the warm sausages with chilled Dijon sauce. Enjoy!

6Ethiopian-Style Chicken with Cauliflower

Preparation Time: 30 minutes

Servings: 6

Nutrition: 234 Calories; 13g Fat; 7g Carbs; 24g Protein; 4g Sugars; 1g Fiber

Ingredients:

2 handful fresh Italian parsleys, roughly chopped

½ cup fresh chopped chives

2 sprigs thyme

6 chicken drumsticks

1 ½ small-sized head cauliflower, broken into large-sized florets

For the Berbere Spice Rub Mix:

2 teaspoons mustard powder

1/3 teaspoon porcini powder

1 ½ teaspoons berbere spice

1/3teaspoon sweet paprika

1/2 teaspoon shallot powder

1teaspoon granulated garlic

1 teaspoon freshly cracked pink peppercorns

1/2 teaspoon sea salt

Directions:

Simply combine all items for the berbere spice rub mix. After that, coat the chicken drumsticks with this rub mix on all sides. Transfer them to the baking dish.

Now, lower the cauliflower onto the chicken drumsticks. Add thyme, chives and Italian parsley and spritz everything with a pan spray. Transfer the baking dish to the preheated Air Fryer. Next step, set the timer for 28 minutes; roast at 355 degrees F, turning occasionally. Bon appétit!

6Herbed Parmesan Chicken Breasts

Preparation Time: 35 minutes
Servings: 6
Nutrition: 231 Calories; 6g Fat; 9g Carbs; 33g Protein; 1g Sugars; 2g Fiber
Ingredients:
3 boneless and skinless chicken breasts, cut into small pieces
1/3 cup cooking wine (such as Sauvignon Blanc
1teaspoon fresh sage leaves, minced
1 teaspoon freshly cracked black pepper
1/3 cup Parmigiano-Reggiano cheese, freshly grated
3 cloves garlic, minced
2 tablespoons olive oil
1 teaspoon seasoned salt
1 teaspoon fresh rosemary leaves, minced
Directions:
Warm the oil in a sauté pan over a moderate flame. Then, sauté the garlic until just fragrant. Next, remove the pan from the heat; pour in the cooking wine. Add the seasonings and toss until everything is well combined. Pour this mixture into a lightly-oiled baking dish.
Toss in the pieces of chicken breasts; roast in the preheated Air Fryer at 325 degrees F for 32 minutes. Scatter grated cheese over the chicken and serve on individual plates.

MEAT

Basil Meatloaf with Parmesan

Preparation Time: 40 minutes
Servings: 5
Ingredients:
1 cup tomato basil sauce, divided in 2
1 ½ lb ground beef
1 ¼ cup diced onion
2 tbsp minced garlic
2 tbsp minced ginger
½ cup breadcrumbs
½ cup grated Parmesan cheese
Salt and black pepper to taste to season
2 tsp cayenne pepper
½ tsp dried basil
⅓ cup chopped parsley
2 egg whites
Directions:
Preheat the Air Fryer to 360 F. In a bowl, add the beef, half of the tomato sauce, onion, garlic, ginger, breadcrumbs, cheese, salt, pepper, cayenne pepper, dried basil, parsley, and egg whites; mix well.
Grease an 8 or 10-inch pan with cooking spray and scoop the meat mixture into it. Shape the meat into the pan while pressing firmly. Brush the remaining tomato sauce onto meat. Place the pan in the fryer basket and close the Air Fryer; cook for 25 minutes. After 15 minutes, open the fryer, and use a meat thermometer to ensure the meat has reached 160 F internally. If not, cook further for 5 minutes. Remove the pan, drain any excess liquid and fat. Let meatloaf cool for 20 minutes before slicing. Serve with a side of sautéed green beans.

Homemade Beef Liver Soufflé

Preparation Time: 40 minutes
Servings: 4
Ingredients:
½ lb of beef liver
3 eggs
3 oz buns
1 cup warm milk
Salt and black pepper to taste
Directions:
Cut the liver in slices and put it in the fridge for 15 minutes. Divide the buns into pieces and soak them in milk for 10 minutes. Put the liver in a blender, and add the yolks, the bread mixture, and the spices. Grind the components and stuff in the ramekins. Line the ramekins in the Air Fryer's basket; cook for 20 minutes at 350 F.

Rib Eye Steak with Avocado Sauce

Preparation Time: 35 minutes
Servings: 4
Ingredients:
1 ½ lb rib eye steak
2 tsp olive oil

1 tbsp chipotle chili pepper
Salt and black pepper to taste
1 avocado, diced
Juice from ½ lime

Directions:

Place the steak on a chopping board. Pour the olive oil over and sprinkle with the chipotle pepper, salt, and black pepper. Use your hands to rub the spices on the meat. Leave it to sit and marinate for 10 minutes.

Preheat the Air Fryer to 400 F. Pull out the fryer basket and place the meat inside. Slide it back into the Air Fryer and cook for 14 minutes. Turn the steak and continue cooking for 6 minutes. Remove the steak, cover with foil, and let it sit for 5 minutes before slicing.

Meanwhile, prepare the avocado salsa by mashing the avocado with potato mash. Add in the lime juice and mix until smooth. Taste, adjust the seasoning, slice and serve with salsa.

Hot Flank Steaks with Roasted Peanuts

Preparation Time: 25 minutes
Servings: 3 to 4
Ingredients:

2 lb flank steaks, cut in long strips
2 tbsp fish sauce
2 tbsp soy sauce
2 tbsp sugar
2 tbsp ground garlic
2 tbsp ground ginger
2 tsp hot sauce
1 cup chopped cilantro, divided into two
½ cup roasted peanuts, chopped

Directions:

Preheat the Air Fryer to 400 F. In a zipper bag, add the beef, fish sauce, swerve sweetener, garlic, soy sauce, ginger, half of the cilantro, and hot sauce. Zip the bag and massage the **Ingredients:** with your hands to mix well.

Open the bag, remove the beef, shake off the excess marinade and place the beef strips in the fryer basket in a single layer; avoid overlapping. Close the Air Fryer and cook for 5 minutes. Turn the beef and cook further for 5 minutes. Dish the cooked meat in a serving platter, garnish with the peanuts and the remaining cilantro.

Authentic Wiener Beef Schnitzel

Preparation Time: 25 minutes
Servings: 4
Ingredients:

4 beef schnitzel cutlets
½ cup flour
2 eggs, beaten
Salt and black pepper
1 cup breadcrumbs

Directions:

Coat the cutlets in flour and shake off any excess. Dip the coated cutlets into the beaten egg. Sprinkle with salt and black pepper. Then dip into the crumbs and to coat well. Spray them generously with oil and cook for 10 minutes at 360 F, turning once halfway through.

Dreamy Beef Steak with Rice, Broccoli and Green Beans

Preparation Time: 40 minutes
Servings: 2
Ingredients:
Beef:
1 lb beef steak,
Salt and black pepper to taste to season
Fried Rice:
2 ½ cups rice
1 ½ tbsp. soy sauce
2 tsp sesame oil
2 tsp minced ginger
2 tsp vinegar
1 clove garlic, minced
¼ cup chopped broccoli
¼ cup green beans
Directions:
Put the beef on a chopping board and use a knife to cut it in 2-inch strips. Add the beef to a bowl, sprinkle with pepper and salt, and mix it with a spoon. Let it sit for 10 minutes. Preheat the Air Fryer to 400 F. Add the beef to the fryer basket, and cook for 5 minutes. Turn the beef strips with kitchen tongs and cook further for 3 minutes.
Once ready, remove the beef to a safe-oven dish that fits in the fryer's basket. Add the rice, broccoli, green beans, garlic, ginger, sesame oil, vinegar and soy sauce. Mix evenly using a spoon. Place the dish in the fryer basket, close, and cook at 370 F for 10 minutes. Open the Air Fryer, mix the rice well, and cook for 4 minutes; season with salt and pepper. Dish the rice into serving bowls and serve with hot sauce.

Mustard Pork Chops with Lemon Zest

Preparation Time: 25 minutes
Servings: 3
Ingredients:
3 lean pork chops
Salt and black pepper to taste to season
2 eggs, cracked into a bowl
1 tbsp water
1 cup breadcrumbs
½ tsp garlic powder
3 tsp paprika
1 ½ tsp oregano
½ tsp cayenne pepper
¼ tsp dry mustard
1 lemon, zested
Directions:
Put the pork chops on a chopping board and use a knife to trim off any excess fat. Add the water to the eggs and whisk; set aside. In another bowl, add the breadcrumbs, salt, pepper, garlic powder, paprika, oregano, cayenne pepper, lemon zest, and dry mustard. Use a fork to mix evenly.
Preheat the Air Fryer to 380 F and grease the basket with cooking spray. In the egg mixture, dip each pork chop and then in the breadcrumb mixture. Place the breaded chops in the fryer. Don't

spray with cooking spray. The fat in the chops will be enough oil to cook them. Close the Air Fryer and cook for 12 minutes.
Flip to other side and cook for another 5 minutes.
Once ready, place the chops on a chopping board to rest for 3 minutes before slicing and serving. Serve with a side of vegetable fries.

Herbed Beef Roast

Preparation Time: 50 minutes
Servings: 2
Ingredients:
2 tsp olive oil
1 lb beef Roast
½ tsp dried rosemary
½ tsp dried thyme
½ tsp dried oregano
Salt and black pepper to taste
Directions:
Preheat the Air Fryer to 400 F. Drizzle oil over the beef, and sprinkle with salt, pepper, and herbs. Rub onto the meat with hands. Cook for 45 minutes for medium-rare and 50 minutes for well-done.
Check halfway through, and flip to ensure they cook evenly. Wrap the beef in foil for 10 minutes after cooking to allow the juices to reabsorb into the meat. Slice the beef and serve with a side of steamed asparagus.

Roast Pork Belly with Cumin

Preparation 4 hrs 30 minutes
Servings: 8
Ingredients:
1 ½ lb pork belly
1 ½ tsp garlic powder
1 ½ tsp coriander powder
⅓ tsp salt
1 ½ tsp black pepper
1 ½ dried thyme
1 ½ tsp dried oregano
1 ½ tsp cumin powder
3 cups water
1 lemon, halved
Directions:
Leave the pork to air fry for 3 hours. In a small bowl, add the garlic powder, coriander powder, ½ tsp of salt, black pepper, thyme, oregano, and cumin powder. After the pork is well dried, poke holes all around it using a fork. Smear the oregano rub thoroughly on all sides with your hands and squeeze the lemon juice all over it.
Leave to sit for 5 minutes. Put the pork in the center of the fryer basket and cook for 30 minutes. Turn the pork with the help of two spatulas, increase the temperature to 350 F and continue cooking for 25 minutes.
Once ready, remove it and place it in on a chopping board to sit for 4 minutes before slicing. Serve the pork slices with a side of sautéed asparagus and hot sauce.

Sunday Night Garlic Beef Schnitzel

Preparation Time: 22 minutes
Servings: 1
Ingredients:
2 tbsp olive oil
1 thin beef cutlet
1 egg, beaten
2 oz breadcrumbs
1 tsp paprika
¼ tsp garlic powder
Salt and black pepper to taste
Directions:
Preheat the air fryer to 350 F. Combine olive oil, breadcrumbs, paprika, garlic powder, and salt, in a bowl. Dip the beef in with the egg first, and then coat it with the breadcrumb mixture completely. Line a baking dish with parchment paper and place the breaded meat on it. Cook for 12 minutes. Serve and enjoy.

Meatballs with Parsley and Thyme

Preparation Time: 25 minutes
Servings: 6
Ingredients:
1 small onion, chopped
¾ pound grounded beef
1 tbsp fresh parsley, chopped
½ tbsp fresh thyme leaves, chopped
1 whole egg, beaten
3 tbsp breadcrumbs
Salt and black pepper to taste
Tomato sauce for coating
Directions:
Preheat your Air Fryer to 390 F. In a mixing bowl, mix all the **Ingredients:** except tomato sauce. Roll the mixture into 10-12 balls. Place the balls in your air fryer's cooking basket, and cook for 8 minutes. Add tomato sauce to the balls to coat and cook for 5 minutes at 300 F. Gently stir and enjoy!

Garlic Lamb Chops with Thyme

Preparation Time: 30 minutes
Servings: 4
Ingredients:
4 lamb chops
1 garlic clove, peeled
1 tbsp plus
2 tsp olive oil
½ tbsp oregano
½ tbsp thyme
½ tsp salt
¼ tsp black pepper
Directions:
Preheat the air fryer to 390 F. Coat the garlic clove with 1 tsp. of olive oil and place it in the air fryer for 10 minutes. Meanwhile, mix the herbs and seasonings with the remaining olive oil.

Using a towel or a mitten, squeeze the hot roasted garlic clove into the herb mixture and stir to combine. Coat the lamb chops with the mixture well, and place in the air fryer. Cook for 8 to 12 minutes.

Ginger Rack Rib Steak

Preparation Time: 35 minutes
Servings: 2
Ingredients:
1 rack rib steak
Salt to season
1 tsp white pepper
1 tsp garlic powder
½ tsp red pepper flakes
1 tsp ginger powder
1 cup Hot sauce
Directions:
Preheat the Air Fryer to 360 F. Place the rib rack on a flat surface and pat dry using a paper towel. Season the ribs with salt, garlic, ginger, white pepper, and red pepper flakes.
Place the ribs in the fryer's basket and cook for 15 minutes. Turn the ribs with kitchen tongs and cook further for 15 minutes. Remove the ribs onto a chopping board and let sit for 3 minutes before slicing. Plate and drizzle hot sauce over and serve.

Bacon-Wrapped Stuffed Pork Tenderloin

Preparation Time: 40 minutes
Servings: 4
Ingredients:
16 bacon slices
16 oz pork tenderloin
Salt and black pepper to taste to season
1 cup spinach
3 oz cream cheese
1 small onion, sliced
1 tbsp olive oil
1 clove garlic, minced
½ tsp dried thyme
½ tsp dried rosemary
Directions:
Place the tenderloin on a chopping board, cover it with a plastic wrap and pound it using a kitchen hammer to a 2-inches flat and square piece. Trim the uneven sides with a knife to have a perfect square. Set aside on a flat plate. On the same chopping board, place and weave the bacon slices into a square of the size of the pork.
Place the pork on the bacon weave and set aside. Put a skillet over medium heat on a stovetop, add olive oil, onions, and garlic; sauté until transparent. Add the spinach, ½ tsp rosemary, ½ tsp thyme, a bit of salt, and pepper.
Stir with a spoon and allow the spinach to wilt. Stir in the cream cheese, until the mixture is even. Turn off.
Preheat the Air Fryer to 360 F. Spoon and spread the spinach mixture onto the pork loin. Roll up the bacon and pork over the spinach stuffing. Secure the ends with as many toothpicks as necessary. Season with more salt and pepper. Place it in the fryer basket and cook for 15 minutes. Flip to other side and cook for another 5 minutes.

Once ready, remove to a clean chopping board. Let sit for 4 minutes before slicing. Serve with steamed veggies.

American-Style Beef Burgers

Preparation Time: 255 minutes
Servings: 4
Ingredients:
Beef:
1 ½ lb ground beef
Salt and black pepper to taste to season
¼ tsp liquid smoke
2 tsp onion powder
1 tsp garlic powder
1 ½ tbsp worcestershire sauce
Burgers:
4 buns
4 trimmed lettuce leaves
4 tbsp mayonnaise
1 large tomato, sliced
4 slices Cheddar cheese
Directions:
Preheat the Air Fryer to 370 F. In a bowl, combine the beef, salt, pepper, liquid smoke, onion powder, garlic powder and Worcestershire sauce using your hands. Form 3 to 4 patties out of the mixture. Place the patties in the fryer basket making sure to leave enough space between them. Ideally, work with two patties at a time. Close the Air Fryer and cook for 10 minutes. Turn the beef with kitchen tongs, reduce the temperature to 350 F, and cook further for 5 minutes. Remove the patties onto a plate. Assemble burgers with the lettuce, mayonnaise, sliced cheese, and sliced tomato.

Basil Pork Patties with Cheddar

Preparation Time: 35 minutes
Servings: 2
Ingredients:
½ lb ground pork
1 medium onion, chopped
1 tbsp mixed herbs
2 tsp garlic powder
1 tsp dried basil
1 tbsp tomato puree
1 tsp mustard
Salt and black pepper to taste
2 bread buns, halved
Assembling:
1 large onion, sliced in 2-inch rings
1 large tomato, sliced in 2-inch rings
2 small lettuce leaves, cleaned
4 slices Cheddar cheese
Directions:
In a bowl, add the minced pork, chopped onion, mixed herbs, garlic powder, dried basil, tomato puree, mustard, salt, and pepper. Use hands to mix evenly. Form two patties out of the mixture and place them on a flat plate.

Preheat the Air Fryer to 370 F. Place the pork patties in the fryer basket, and cook for 15 minutes. Slide out the basket and turn the patties with a spatula. Reduce the temperature to 350 F and cook for 5 minutes.

Once ready, remove them onto a plate and start assembling the burger. Place two halves of the bun on a clean flat surface. Add the lettuce in both, then a patty each, followed by an onion ring each, a tomato ring each, and then 2 slices of cheddar cheese each. Cover the buns with their other halves. Serve with ketchup and french fries.

Tasty Sausage Bacon Rolls

Preparation Time: 1 hour 44 minutes
Servings: 4
Ingredients:
Sausage:
8 bacon strips
8 pork sausages
Relish:
8 large tomatoes
1 clove garlic, peeled
1 small onion, peeled
3 tbsp chopped parsley
A pinch of salt
A pinch of pepper
2 tbsp sugar
1 tsp smoked paprika
1 tbsp white wine vinegar
Directions:
Start with the relish; add the tomatoes, garlic, and onion in a food processor. Blitz them for 10 seconds until the mixture is pulpy. Pour the pulp into a saucepan, add the vinegar, salt, pepper, and place it over medium heat.

Bring to simmer for 10 minutes; add the paprika and sugar. Stir with a spoon and simmer for 10 minutes until pulpy and thick. Turn off the heat, transfer the relish to a bowl and chill it for an hour. In 30 minutes after putting the relish in the refrigerator, move on to the sausages. Wrap each sausage with a bacon strip neatly and stick in a bamboo skewer at the end of the sausage to secure the bacon ends.

Open the Air Fryer, place 3 to 4 wrapped sausages in the fryer basket and cook for 12 minutes at 350 F. Ensure that the bacon is golden and crispy before removing them. Repeat the cooking process for the remaining wrapped sausages. Remove the relish from the refrigerator. Serve the sausages and relish with turnip mash.

Delicious Beef Roast with Red Potatoes

Preparation Time: 25 minutes
Servings: 3
Ingredients:
2 tbsp olive oil
4 pound top round roast beef
1 tsp salt
¼ tsp fresh ground black pepper
1 tsp dried thyme
½ tsp fresh rosemary, chopped
3 pounds red potatoes, halved
Olive oil, black pepper and salt for garnish

Directions:
Preheat your Air Fryer to 360 F. In a small bowl, mix rosemary, salt, pepper and thyme; rub oil onto beef. Season with the spice mixture. Place the prepared meat in your Air Fryer's cooking basket and cook for 20 minutes.
Give the meat a turn and add potatoes, more pepper and oil. Cook for 20 minutes more. Take the steak out and set aside to cool for 10 minutes. Cook the potatoes in your Air Fryer for 10 more minutes at 400 F. Serve hot.

Beef, Mushrooms and Noodles Dish

Preparation Time: 35 minutes
Servings: 5
Ingredients:
1½ pounds beef steak
1 package egg noodles, cooked
1 ounce dry onion soup mix
1 can (15 oz cream mushroom soup
2 cups mushrooms, sliced
1 whole onion, chopped
½ cup beef broth
3 garlic cloves, minced?
Directions:
Preheat your Air Fryer to 360 F. Drizzle onion soup mix all over the meat. In a mixing bowl, mix the sauce, garlic cloves, beef broth, chopped onion, sliced mushrooms and mushroom soup. Top the meat with the prepared sauce mixture. Place the prepared meat in the air fryer's cooking basket and cook for 25 minutes. Serve with cooked egg noodles.

Lemongrass Pork Chops

Preparation Time: 2 hrs 20 minutes
Servings: 3
Ingredients:
3 slices pork chops
2 garlic cloves, minced
1 ½ tbsp sugar
4 stalks lemongrass, trimmed and chopped
2 shallots, chopped
2 tbsp olive oil
1 ¼ tsp soy sauce
1 ¼ tsp fish sauce
1 ½ tsp black pepper
Directions:
In a bowl, add the garlic, sugar, lemongrass, shallots, olive oil, soy sauce, fish sauce, and black pepper; mix well. Add the pork chops, coat them with the mixture and allow to marinate for around 2 hours to get nice and savory.
Preheat the Air Fryer to 400 F. Cooking in 2 to 3 batches, remove and shake each pork chop from the marinade and place it in the fryer basket. Cook it for 7 minutes. Turn the pork chops with kitchen tongs and cook further for 5 minutes. Remove the chops and serve with a side of sautéed asparagus.

Effortless Beef Schnitzel

Preparation Time: 25 minutes
Servings: 2
Ingredients:
2 tbsp vegetable oil
2 oz breadcrumbs
1 whole egg, whisked
1 thin beef schnitzel, cut into strips
1 whole lemon
Directions:
Preheat your fryer to 356 F. In a bowl, add breadcrumbs and oil and stir well to get a loose mixture. Dip schnitzel in egg, then dip in breadcrumbs coat well. Place the prepared schnitzel your Air Fryer's cooking basket and cook for 12 minutes. Serve with a drizzle of lemon juice.

BBQ Pork Ribs

Preparation Time: 5 hrs 30 minutes
Servings: 2 to 3
Ingredients:
1 lb pork ribs
1 tsp soy sauce
Salt and black pepper to taste
1 tsp oregano
1 tbsp + 1 tbsp maple syrup
3 tbsp barbecue sauce
2 cloves garlic, minced
1 tbsp cayenne pepper
1 tsp sesame oil
Directions:
Put the chops on a chopping board and use a knife to cut them into smaller pieces of desired sizes. Put them in a mixing bowl, add the soy sauce, salt, pepper, oregano, one tablespoon of maple syrup, barbecue sauce, garlic, cayenne pepper, and sesame oil. Mix well and place the pork in the fridge to marinate in the spices for 5 hours.
Preheat the Air Fryer to 350 F. Open the Air Fryer and place the ribs in the fryer basket. Slide the fryer basket in and cook for 15 minutes. Open the Air fryer, turn the ribs using tongs, apply the remaining maple syrup with a brush, close the Air Fryer, and continue cooking for 10 minutes.

Homemade Beef Stroganoff

Preparation Time: 20 minutes
Servings: 3
Ingredients:
1 pound thin steak
4 tbsp butter
1 whole onion, chopped
1 cup sour cream
8 oz mushrooms, sliced
4 cups beef broth
16 oz egg noodles, cooked

Directions:

Preheat your Air Fryer to 400 F. Using a microwave proof bowl, melt butter in a microwave oven. In a mixing bowl, mix the melted butter, sliced mushrooms, cream, onion, and beef broth. Pour the mixture over steak and set aside for 10 minutes. Place the marinated beef in your fryer's cooking basket, and cook for 10 minutes. Serve with cooked egg noodles and enjoy!

Hot Pork Skewers

Preparation Time: 1 hour 20 minutes
Servings: 3 to 4
Ingredients:

1 lb pork steak, cut in cubes
¼ cup soy sauce
2 tsp smoked paprika
1 tsp powdered chili
1 tsp garlic salt
1 tsp red chili flakes
1 tbsp white wine vinegar
3 tbsp steak sauce
Skewing:
1 green pepper, cut in cubes
1 red pepper, cut in cubes
1 yellow squash, seeded and cut in cubes
1 green squash, seeded and cut in cubes
Salt and black pepper to taste to season

Directions:

In a mixing bowl, add the pork cubes, soy sauce, smoked paprika, powdered chili, garlic salt, red chili flakes, white wine vinegar, and steak sauce. Mix them using a ladle. Refrigerate to marinate them for 1 hour.

After one hour, remove the marinated pork from the fridge and preheat the Air Fryer to 370 F. On each skewer, stick the pork cubes and vegetables in the order that you prefer. Have fun doing this. Once the pork cubes and vegetables are finished, arrange the skewers in the fryer basket and grill them for 8 minutes. You can do them in batches. Once ready, remove them onto the serving platter and serve with salad.

Pork Rack with Macadamia Nuts

Preparation Time: 50minutes
Servings: 2 to 3
Ingredients:

1 lb rack of pork
2 tbsp olive oil
1 clove garlic, minced
Salt and black pepper to taste
1 cup chopped macadamia nuts
1 tbsp breadcrumbs
1 egg, beaten in a bowl
1 tbsp rosemary, chopped

Directions:

Add the olive oil and garlic to a bowl. Mix vigorously with a spoon to make garlic oil. Place the rack of pork on a chopping board and brush it with the garlic oil using a brush. Sprinkle with salt and pepper.

Preheat the Air Fryer to 250 F. In a bowl, add breadcrumbs, nuts, and rosemary. Mix with a spoon and set aside. Brush the meat with the egg on all sides and sprinkle the nut mixture generously over the pork. Press with hands. Put the coated pork in the fryer basket, close and roast for 30 minutes.

Increase the temperature to 390 F and cook further for 5 minutes. Once ready, remove the meat onto a chopping board. Allow a sitting time of 10 minutes before slicing. Serve with a side of parsnip fries and tomato dip.

Sweet Marinaded Pork Chops

Preparation Time:15 minutes
Servings: 3
Ingredients:
3 pork chops, ½-inch thick
Salt and black pepper to taste to season
1 tbsp maple syrup
1 ½ tbsp minced garlic
3 tbsp mustard
Directions:
In a bowl, add maple syrup, garlic, mustard, salt, and pepper; mix well. Add the pork and toss it in the mustard sauce to coat well. Slide out the fryer basket and place the chops in the basket; cook at 350 F for 6 minutes.

Open the Air Fryer and flip the pork with a spatula and cook further for 6 minutes. Once ready, remove them onto a serving platter and serve with a side of steamed asparagus.

Savory Pulled Pork with Cheddar and Bacon

Preparation Time: 50 minutes
Servings: 2
Ingredients:
½ pork steak
1 tsp steak seasoning
Salt and black pepper to taste
5 thick bacon slices, chopped
1 cup grated Cheddar cheese
½ tbsp worcestershire sauce
2 bread buns, halved
Directions:
Preheat the Air Fryer to 400 F. Place the pork steak in a plate and season with pepper, salt, and the steak seasoning. Pat it with your hands. Slide out the fryer basket and place the pork in it. Grill for 15 minutes, turn using tongs, slide the fryer in and continue cooking for 6 minutes.

Once ready, remove the steak onto a chopping board and use two forks to shred the pork into small pieces. Place the chopped bacon in a small heatproof bowl and place the bowl in the fryer's basket.

Close the Air Fryer and cook the bacon at 370 F for 10 minutes. Remove the bacon into a bigger heatproof bowl, add the pulled pork, Worcestershire sauce, and the cheddar cheese. Season with salt and pepper.

Place the bowl in the fryer basket and cook at 350 for 4 minutes. Slide out the fryer basket, stir the mixture with a spoon, slide the fryer basket back in and cook further for 1 minute. Spoon to scoop the meat into the halved buns and serve with a cheese or tomato dip.

Teriyaki Pork Ribs with Tomato Sauce

Preparation Time: 20 minutes
Servings: 3
Ingredients:
1 pound pork ribs
1 tsp salt
1 tsp pepper
1 tbsp sugar
1 tsp ginger juice
1 tsp five-spice powder
1 tbsp teriyaki sauce
1 tbsp light soy sauce
1 garlic clove, minced
2 tbsp honey
1 tbsp water
1 tbsp tomato sauce
Directions:
In a bowl, mix pepper, sugar, five-spice powder, salt, ginger juice, teriyaki sauce. Add pork ribs to the marinade and let marinate for 2 hours. Preheat your Air Fryer to 350 F.
Add pork ribs to your Air Fryer's cooking basket and cook for 8 minutes. In a separate mixing bowl, mix soy sauce, garlic, honey, water, tomato sauce. Over medium heat, add oil and garlic in a pan and fry for 30 seconds. Add fried pork ribs and pour the prepared sauce. Stir-fry for a few minutes, serve and enjoy!

Tamarind Pork Chops with Caramelized Potatoes

Preparation Time: 45 minutes
Servings: 4
Ingredients:
2 tbsp tamarind paste
2 whole caramelized potatoes
1 tbsp garlic, minced
½ cup green mole sauce
3 tbsp corn syrup
1 tbsp olive oil
2 tbsp molasses
4 tbsp southwest seasoning
2 tbsp ketchup
4 pork chops
2 tbsp water
Directions:
Preheat your Air Fryer to 350 F. In a bowl, mix all the **Ingredients:** except potatoes, pork chops and mole sauce.
Let the pork chops marinate in the mixture for 30 minutes. Place pork chops to your Air Fryer's cooking basket and cook for 25 minutes. Serve with caramelized potatoes and mole sauce.

Oyster Beef Steak with Broccoli

Preparation Time: 35 minutes
Servings: 4
Ingredients:
¾ pound circular beef steak, cut into strips

1 pound broccoli, cut into florets
⅓ cup oyster sauce
2 tbsp sesame oil
⅓ cup sherry
1 tsp soy sauce
1 tsp white sugar
1 tsp cornstarch
1 tbsp olive oil
1 garlic clove, minced

Directions:

In a bowl, mix cornstarch, sherry, oyster sauce, sesame oil, soy sauce, sugar and beef steaks. Set aside for 45 minutes. Add garlic, oil and ginger to the steaks. Place the steaks in your air fryer's cooking basket and cook for

Cheesy Stuffed Peppers with Ground Pork

Preparation Time: 30 minutes
Servings: 3
Nutrition: 425 Calories; 29g Fat; 5g Carbs; 33g Protein; 2g Sugars; 2g Fiber

Ingredients:

3 bell peppers, stems and seeds removed
1 tablespoon olive oil
3 scallions, chopped
1 teaspoon fresh garlic, minced
12 ounces lean pork, ground
1/2 teaspoon sea salt
1/2 teaspoon black pepper
1 tablespoon fish sauce
2 ripe tomatoes, pureed
3 ounces Monterey Jack cheese, grated

Directions:

Cook the peppers in boiling salted water for 4 minutes
In a nonstick skillet, heat the olive oil over medium heat. Then, sauté the scallions and garlic until tender and fragrant.
Stir in the ground pork and continue sautéing until the pork has browned; drain off the excess fat.
Add the salt, black pepper, fish sauce, and 1 pureed tomato; give it a good stir.
Divide the filling among the bell peppers. Arrange the peppers in a baking dish lightly greased with cooking oil. Place the remaining tomato puree around the peppers.
Bake in the preheated Air Fryer at 380 degrees F for 13 minutes. Top with grated cheese and bake another 6 minutes. Serve warm and enjoy!

Mexican Salsa Boston Butt

Preparation Time: 35 minutes
Servings: 4
Nutrition: 374 Calories; 21g Fat; 6g Carbs; 29g Protein; 7g Sugars; 9g Fiber

Ingredients:

1 pound Boston butt, thinly sliced across the grain into 2-inch-long strips
1/2 teaspoon red pepper flakes, crushed
Sea salt and ground black pepper, to taste
1/2 pound tomatillos, chopped
1 small-sized onion, chopped

2 chili peppers, chopped
2 cloves garlic
2 tablespoons fresh cilantro, chopped
1 tablespoon olive oil
1 teaspoon sea salt

Directions:

Rub the Boston butt with red pepper, salt, and black pepper. Spritz the bottom of the cooking basket with a nonstick cooking spray.

Roast the Boston butt in the preheated Air Fryer at 390 degrees F for 10 minutes. Shake the basket and cook another 10 minutes.

While the pork is roasting, make the salsa.

Blend the remaining **Ingredients:** until smooth and uniform. Transfer the mixture to a saucepan and add 1 cup of water.

Bring to a boil; reduce the heat and simmer for 8 to 12 minutes. Serve the roasted pork with the salsa verde on the side. Enjoy!

Pork with Buttery Broccoli

Preparation Time: 30 minutes
Servings: 4
Nutrition: 346 Calories; 11g Fat; 4g Carbs; 32g Protein; 1g Sugars; 1g Fiber

Ingredients:

1 ½ pounds blade steaks skinless, boneless
Kosher salt and ground black pepper, to taste
2 garlic cloves, crushed
2 tablespoons coconut aminos
1 tablespoon oyster sauce
2 tablespoon lemon juice
1 pound broccoli, broken into florets
2 tablespoons butter, melted
1 teaspoon dried dill weed
2 tablespoons sunflower seeds, lightly toasted

Directions:

Start by preheating your Air Fryer to 385 degrees F. Spritz the bottom and sides of the cooking basket with cooking spray.

Now, season the pork with salt and black pepper. Add the garlic, coconut aminos, oyster sauce, and lemon juice.

Cook for 20 minutes; turning over halfway through the cooking time.

Toss the broccoli with the melted butter and dill. Add the broccoli to the cooking basket and cook at 400 degrees F for 6 minutes, shaking the basket periodically.

Serve the warm pork with broccoli and garnish with sunflower seeds. Bon appétit!

Sloppy Joes with a Twist

Preparation Time: 45 minutes
Servings: 4
Nutrition: 571 Calories; 41g Fat; 3g Carbs; 31g Protein; 7g Sugars; 9g Fiber

Ingredients:

1 tablespoon olive oil
1 shallot, chopped
2 garlic cloves, minced
1 bell pepper, chopped

1 pound ground pork
1 ripe medium-sized tomato, pureed
1 tablespoon poultry seasoning blend
Dash ground allspice
Keto Buns:
1/3 cup ricotta cheese, crumbled
2/3 cup part skim mozzarella cheese, shredded
1 egg
1/3 cup coconut flour
1/2 cup almond flour
1 teaspoon baking soda
1 ½ tablespoons plain whey protein isolate

Directions:

Start by preheating your Air Fryer to 390 degrees F. Heat the olive oil for a few minutes.
Once hot, sauté the shallots until just tender. Add the garlic and bell pepper; cook for 4 minutes more or until they are aromatic.
Add the ground pork and cook for 5 minutes more, crumbling with a fork. Next step, stir in the pureed tomatoes and spices. Decrease the temperature to 365 degrees F and cook another 10 minutes. Reserve.
To make the keto buns, microwave the cheese for 1 minute 30 seconds, stirring twice. Add the cheese to the bowl of a food processor and blend well. Fold in the egg and mix again.
Add in the flour, baking soda, and plain whey protein isolate; blend again. Scrape the batter onto the center of a lightly greased cling film.
Form the dough into a disk and transfer to your freezer to cool; cut into 4 pieces and transfer to a parchment-lined baking pan (make sure to grease your hands). Bake in the preheated oven at 400 degrees F for about 14 minutes.
Spoon the meat mixture into keto buns and transfer them to the cooking basket. Cook for 7 minutes or until thoroughly warmed.

Spicy and Saucy Pork Sirloin

Preparation Time: 55 minutes
Servings: 3
Nutrition: 426 Calories; 26g Fat; 1g Carbs; 44g Protein; 8g Sugars; 4g Fiber

Ingredients:

2 teaspoons peanut oil
1 ½ pounds pork sirloin
Coarse sea salt and ground black pepper, to taste
1 tablespoon smoked paprika
1/4 cup prepared salsa sauce

Directions:

Start by preheating your Air Fryer to 360 degrees F.
Drizzle the oil all over the pork sirloin. Sprinkle with salt, black pepper, and paprika.
Cook for 50 minutes in the preheated Air Fryer.
Remove the roast from the Air Fryer and shred with two forks. Mix in the salsa sauce. Enjoy!

French-Style Smothered Pork Chops

Preparation Time: 20 minutes
Servings: 4
Nutrition: 307 Calories; 5g Fat; 7g Carbs; 39g Protein; 9g Sugars; 4g Fiber

Ingredients:

2 tablespoons coconut aminos

2 tablespoons French wine
2 tablespoons rice vinegar
1 pound pork loin center rib chops, bone-in
1 teaspoon Herbes de Provence
Celtic salt and ground black pepper, to taste
1 tablespoon Dijon mustard

Directions:

Thoroughly combine the coconut aminos, wine, and vinegar; add the pork and let it marinate for 1 hour in the refrigerator.

Sprinkle the pork chops with Herbes de Provence, salt, and black pepper. Spread the mustard, all over the pork chops.

Cook in the preheated Air Fryer at 400 degrees F for 12 minutes. Serve warm with mashed potatoes if desired.

Authentic Pakistani Seekh Kebabs

Preparation Time: 25 minutes
Servings: 3
Nutrition: 456 Calories; 37g Fat; 1g Carbs; 21g Protein; 5g Sugars; 6g Fiber

Ingredients:

1 pound lean pork, ground
1 onion, chopped
1 garlic clove, smashed
1 Thai bird chili, deveined and finely chopped
1 teaspoon mustard
1 teaspoon coriander seed, ground
1/2 teaspoon cumin powder
Salt and ground black pepper, to taste
6 tablespoons parmesan cheese, grated

Directions:

Mix all **Ingredients:** using your hands. Knead until everything is well incorporated.

Shape the meat mixture around flat skewers (sausage shapes).

Cook at 365 degrees F for 11 to 12 minutes, turning them over once or twice. Work in batches. Serve!

Spicy Pork Sausage with Eggs

Preparation Time: 24 minutes
Servings: 6
Nutrition: 468 Calories; 39g Fat; 6g Carbs; 26g Protein; 3g Sugars; 7g Fiber

Ingredients:

1 green bell pepper, seeded and thinly sliced
6 medium-sized eggs
1 Habanero pepper, seeded and minced
1/2 teaspoon sea salt
2 teaspoons fennel seeds
1 red bell pepper, seeded and thinly sliced
1 teaspoon tarragon
1/2 teaspoon freshly cracked black pepper
6 pork sausages

Directions:

Place the sausages and all peppers in the Air Fryer cooking basket. Cook at 335 degrees F for 9 minutes.

Divide the eggs among 6 ramekins; sprinkle each egg with the seasonings.

Cook for 11 more minutes at 395 degrees F. Serve warm with sausages. Bon appétit!

Pork Tenderloin with Garden Vegetables

Preparation Time: 20 minutes
Servings: 2
Nutrition: 268 Calories; 7g Fat; 5g Carbs; 41g Protein; 6g Sugars; 8g Fiber
Ingredients:

½ cup cream of onion soup
½ bell pepper, seeded and diced
Fine sea salt and black pepper, to taste
1/3 cup celery, chopped
1/2 pound pork tenderloin, diced
1/3 cup onions, chopped
2 teaspoons cayenne pepper
2 garlic cloves, halved

Directions:

Begin by preheating your air fryer to 385 degrees F.

Add all **Ingredients:** to a baking dish that is previously greased with a thin layer of canola oil; cook about 5 minutes.

Gently stir the **Ingredients:** and cook an additional 12 minutes. Bon appétit!

Peppery Pork Roast with Herbs

Preparation Time: 30 minutes
Servings: 6
Nutrition: 241 Calories; 14g Fat; 3g Carbs; 22g Protein; 3g Sugars; 8g Fiber
Ingredients:

1 tablespoon olive oil
1 pound pork loin
1 teaspoon dried basil
1/2 teaspoon dried oregano
¼ teaspoon crushed red pepper flakes
1 teaspoon dried thyme
1/4 teaspoon freshly grated nutmeg
Sea salt flakes and freshly ground black pepper, to taste
1 Pimento chili pepper, deveined and chopped
1 Yellow wax pepper, deveined and chopped
1 bell pepper, deveined and chopped
1 tablespoon peanut butter
1/4 cup beef broth
1/2 tablespoon whole-grain mustard
1 bay leaf

Directions:

Lightly grease the inside of an Air Fryer baking dish with a thin layer of olive oil. Then, cut 8 slit down the center of pork (about 3x3"). Sprinkle with the seasonings and massage them into the meat to evenly distribute

Then, tuck peppers into the slits and transfer the meat to the Air Fryer baking dish. Scatter remaining peppers around the roast.

In a mixing dish, whisk the peanut butter, beef broth, and mustard; now, pour broth mixture around the roast.
Add the bay leaf and roast the meat for 25 minutes at 390 degrees F; turn the pork over halfway through the roasting time. Bon appétit!

Pork Sausage Meatloaf with Veggies

Preparation Time: 30 minutes
Servings: 6
Nutrition: 282 Calories; 12g Fat; 2g Carbs; 13g Protein; 1g Sugars; 1g Fiber
Ingredients:
Non-stick cooking spray
1 shallot, finely chopped
1 rib celery, finely chopped
2 gloves garlic, minced
1 tablespoon Worcestershire sauce
3/4 pound spicy ground pork sausage
1/4 pound ground turkey
2 sprigs rosemary, leaves only, crushed
1/4 cup minced fresh parsley
1 egg, lightly whisked
3 tablespoons fresh panko
Salt and freshly ground pepper, to your liking
1/3 cup tomato paste
Directions:
Spritz a cast-iron skillet with a cooking spray. Then, sauté the shallots, celery and garlic until just tender and fragrant.
Now, add Worcestershire sauce and both kinds of meat to the sautéed mixture. Remove from the heat. Add the rosemary, parsley, egg, fresh panko, salt, and pepper; mix to combine well.
Transfer the mixture to the baking pan and shape into a loaf. Cover the prepared meatloaf with tomato paste.
Air-fry at 390 degrees F for 25 minutes or until thoroughly warmed.

Egg and Sausage Ramekins Breakfast

Preparation Time: 20 minutes
Servings: 5
Nutrition: 385 Calories; 34g Fat; 77g Carbs; 27g Protein; 1g Sugars; 1g Fiber
Ingredients:
1/2 teaspoon ground black pepper, or more to taste
1/2 teaspoon mustard seeds
10 slices of bacon
1/3 teaspoon fennel seeds
5 eggs
10 pork sausages
1/3 teaspoon kosher salt
Directions:
Divide the sausages and bacon among five ramekins; crack an egg into each ramekin. Sprinkle with seasonings.
Cook for 18 minutes at 345 degrees F or until your eggs reach desired texture.
Serve warm with some extra Dijon mustard and spicy tomato ketchup. Bon appétit!

Pork Chops Romano

Preparation Time: 1 hour 12 minutes
Servings: 4
Nutrition: 466 Calories; 25g Fat; 9g Carbs; 54g Protein; 5g Sugars; 2g Fiber
Ingredients:
3 eggs, well-beaten
1 cup Romano cheese, grated
2 teaspoons mustard powder
1 ½ tablespoons olive oil
1/2 tablespoon soy sauce
2 tablespoons Worcestershire sauce
½ teaspoon dried rosemary
4 large-sized pork chops
½ teaspoon dried thyme
2 teaspoons fennel seeds
Salt and freshly cracked black pepper, to taste
1 teaspoon red pepper flakes, crushed
Directions:
Add the pork chops along with olive oil, soy sauce, Worcestershire sauce, and seasonings to a resealable plastic bag. Allow pork chops to marinate for 50 minutes in your refrigerator.
Next step, dip the pork chops into the beaten eggs; then, coat the pork chops with Romano cheese on both sides. Press the breading firmly into the pork chops.
Cook in the Air Fryer for 18 minutes at 405 degrees F, turning once. Bon appétit!

Rich Meatball and Mushroom Cassoulet

Preparation Time: 41 minutes
Servings: 4
Nutrition: 317 Calories; 22g Fat; 3g Carbs; 21g Protein; 7g Sugars; 1g Fiber
Ingredients:
1/2 cup celery, peeled and grated
1 ½ cup mushrooms, sliced
1/2 cup heavy cream
1/2 cup Monterey Jack cheese, preferably freshly grated
Meatballs:
2 tablespoons pork rinds
12 ounces lean ground pork
1 teaspoon saffron
2 teaspoons fennel seeds
1 medium-sized lees, finely chopped
1/teaspoon dried dill weed
2 small-sized egg
1/2 teaspoon cumin
½ teaspoon fine sea salt
Freshly ground black pepper, to taste
Directions:
Begin by preheating the Air Fryer to 400 degrees F.
In a bowl, mix the **Ingredients:** for the meatballs. Shape the mixture into mini meatballs.
In an Air Fryer baking dish, toss the celery and mushrooms with the cream; cook for 23 minutes in the preheated Air Fryer.

Pause the machine and place the reserved meatballs in a single layer on top of the celery/mushroom mixture.
Top with the grated Monterey Jack cheese; bake for 9 minutes longer. Serve warm.

Mouthwatering Pork Medallions with Creole mustard

Preparation Time: 25 minutes
Servings: 4
Nutrition: 292 Calories; 12g Fat; 9g Carbs; 29g Protein; 1g Sugars; 4g Fiber
Ingredients:
1 pound pork medallions, trimmed and sliced into thick medallions
2 tablespoons Creole mustard
½ tablespoon apple cider vinegar
1 ½ tablespoons extra-virgin olive oil
2 teaspoon cumin seeds, ground
½ teaspoon seasoned salt
1/3 teaspoon freshly cracked black peppercorns, or multi-color peppercorns
Directions:
Toss the pork medallions with all the other items until well coated. Cook in your Air Fryer for 13 minutes at 365 degrees F.
Check for doneness and cook for 4 to 5 minutes longer as needed.
To finish, mound the wilted kale onto a serving plate. Top with the beef medallions and serve immediately.

Spicy Bacon-Pork Pops

Preparation Time: 30 minutes + marinating time
Servings: 6
Nutrition: 572 Calories; 41g Fat; 9g Carbs; 46g Protein; 4g Sugars; 8g Fiber
Ingredients:
1 cup cream of celery soup
1 (15-ouncecan coconut milk, unsweetened
2 tablespoons tamari sauce
1 teaspoon yellow mustard
Salt and freshly ground white pepper, to taste
1/2 teaspoon cayenne pepper
1/2 teaspoon chili powder
1 teaspoon curry powder
2 pounds pork tenderloin, cut into bite-sized cubes
4 ounces bacon, cut into pieces
12 bamboo skewers, soaked in water
Directions:
In a large pot, bring the cream of the celery soup, coconut milk, tamari sauce, mustard, salt, white pepper, cayenne pepper, chili powder, and curry powder to a boil.
Then, reduce the heat to simmer; cook until the sauce is heated through, about 13 minutes.
Add the pork, gently stir, and place in your refrigerator for 2 hours.
Thread the pork onto the skewers, alternating the cubes of meat with the pieces of bacon.
Preheat your Air Fryer to 370 degrees F. Cook for 15 minutes, turning over a couple of times.
Bon appétit!

Classic Ribs with Bell Peppers

Preparation Time: 55 minutes
Servings: 4
Nutrition: 406 Calories; 24g Fat; 10g Carbs; 49g Protein; 6g Sugars; 6g Fiber
Ingredients:
1 pound St. Louis-style pork spareribs, individually cut
1 teaspoon seasoned salt
1/2 teaspoon ground black pepper
1 tablespoon sweet paprika
1/2 teaspoon mustard powder
2 tablespoons sesame oil
4 bell pepper, seeded
Directions:
Toss and rub the spices all over the pork ribs; drizzle with 1 tablespoon of sesame oil.
Cook the pork ribs at 360 degrees F for 15 minutes; flip the ribs and cook an additional 20 minutes or until they are tender inside and crisp on the outside.
Toss the peppers with the remaining 1 tablespoon of oil; season to taste and cook in the preheated Air Fryer at 390 degrees F for 15 minutes.
Serve the warm spareribs with the roasted peppers on the side. Enjoy!

Spicy Pork Curry

Preparation Time: 35 minutes
Servings: 4
Nutrition: 396 Calories; 21g Fat; 9g Carbs; 42g Protein; 6g Sugars; 1g Fiber
Ingredients:
2 cardamom pods, only the seeds, crushed
1 teaspoon fennel seeds
1 teaspoon cumin seeds
1 teaspoon coriander seeds
2 teaspoons peanut oil
2 scallions, chopped
2 garlic cloves, smashed
2 jalapeno peppers, minced
1/2 teaspoon ginger, freshly grated
1 pound pork loin, cut into bite-sized cubes
1 cup coconut milk
1 cup chicken broth
1 teaspoon turmeric powder
1 tablespoon tamarind paste
1 tablespoon fresh lime juice
Directions:
Place the cardamom, fennel, cumin, and coriander seeds in a nonstick skillet over medium-high heat. Stir for 6 minutes until the spices become aromatic and start to brown. Stir frequently to prevent the spices from burning. Set aside.
Preheat your Air Fryer to 370 degrees F. Then, in a baking pan, heat the peanut oil for 2 minutes. Once hot, sauté the scallions for 2 to 3 minutes until tender.
Stir in the garlic, peppers, and ginger; cook an additional minute, stirring frequently. Next, cook the pork for 3 to 4 minutes.
Pour in the coconut milk and broth. Add the reserved seeds, turmeric, and tamarind paste. Let it cook for 15 minutes in the preheated Air Fryer.

Divide between individual bowls; drizzle fresh lime juice over the top and serve immediately.

Nana's Pork Chops with Cilantro

Preparation Time: 22 minutes
Servings: 6
Nutrition: 390 Calories; 23g Fat; 1g Carbs; 42g Protein; 3g Sugars; 2g Fiber
Ingredients:
1/3 cup pork rinds
Roughly chopped fresh cilantro, to taste
2 teaspoons Cajun seasonings
Nonstick cooking spray
2 eggs, beaten
3 tablespoons almond meal
1 teaspoon seasoned salt
Garlic & onion spice blend, to taste
6 pork chops
1/3 teaspoon freshly cracked black pepper
Directions:
Coat the pork chops with Cajun seasonings, salt, pepper, and the spice blend on all sides.
Then, add the almond meal to a plate. In a shallow dish, whisk the egg until pale and smooth. Place the pork rinds in the third bowl.
Dredge each pork piece in the almond meal; then, coat them with the egg; finally, coat them with the pork rinds. Spritz them with cooking spray on both sides.
Now, air-fry pork chops for about 18 minutes at 345 degrees F; make sure to taste for doneness after first 12 minutes of cooking. Lastly, garnish with fresh cilantro. Bon appétit!

Paprika Burgers with Blue Cheese

Preparation Time: 44 minutes
Servings: 6
Nutrition: 493 Calories; 36g Fat; 1g Carbs; 31g Protein; 4g Sugars; 8g Fiber
Ingredients:
1 cup blue cheese, sliced
2 teaspoons dried basil
1 teaspoon smoked paprika
2 pounds ground pork
2 tablespoons tomato puree
2 small-sized onions, peeled and chopped
1/2 teaspoon ground black pepper
3 garlic cloves, minced
1 teaspoon fine sea salt
Directions:
Start by preheating your Air Fryer to 385 degrees F.
In a mixing dish, combine the pork, onion, garlic, tomato puree, and seasonings; mix to combine well.
Form the pork mixture into six patties; cook the burgers for 23 minutes. Pause the machine, turn the temperature to 365 degrees F and cook for 18 more minutes.
Place the prepared burgers on a serving platter; top with blue cheese and serve warm.

Tangy Pork Chops with Vermouth

Preparation Time: 34 minutes
Servings: 5
Nutrition: 400 Calories; 23g Fat; 1g Carbs; 45g Protein; 5g Sugars; 4g Fiber
Ingredients:
5 pork chops
1/3 cup vermouth
1/2 teaspoon paprika
2 sprigs thyme, only leaves, crushed
1/2 teaspoon dried oregano
Fresh parsley, to serve
1 teaspoon garlic salt
½ lemon, cut into wedges
1 teaspoon freshly cracked black pepper
3 tablespoons lemon juice
3 cloves garlic, minced
2 tablespoons canola oil
Directions:
Firstly, heat the canola oil in a sauté pan over a moderate heat. Now, sweat the garlic until just fragrant.
Remove the pan from the heat and pour in the lemon juice and vermouth. Now, throw in the seasonings. Dump the sauce into a baking dish, along with the pork chops.
Tuck the lemon wedges among the pork chops and air-fry for 27 minutes at 345 degrees F. Bon appétit!

French-Style Pork and Pepper Meatloaf

Preparation Time: 35 minutes
Servings: 4
Nutrition: 417 Calories; 21g Fat; 6g Carbs; 39g Protein; 2g Sugars; 9g Fiber
Ingredients:
1 pound pork, ground
1/2 cup parmesan cheese, grated
1 ½ tablespoons green garlic, minced
1½ tablespoon fresh cilantro, minced
1/2 tablespoon fish sauce
1/3 teaspoon dried basil
1 leek, chopped
1 serrano pepper, chopped
2 tablespoons tomato puree
1/2 teaspoons dried thyme
Salt and ground black pepper, to taste
Directions:
Add all **Ingredients:** to a large-sized mixing dish and combine everything using your hands. Then, form a meatloaf using a spatula.
Bake for 23 minutes at 365 degrees F. Afterward, allow your meatloaf to rest for 10 minutes before slicing and serving. Bon appétit!

Ham and Kale Egg Cups

Preparation Time: 20 minutes
Servings: 2
Nutrition: 398 Calories; 18g Fat; 3g Carbs; 61g Protein; 9g Sugars; 1g Fiber
Ingredients:
2 eggs
1/4 teaspoon dried or fresh marjoram
2 teaspoons chili powder
1/3 teaspoon kosher salt
½ cup steamed kale
1/4 teaspoon dried or fresh rosemary
4 pork ham slices
1/3 teaspoon ground black pepper, or more to taste
Directions:
Divide the kale and ham among 2 ramekins; crack an egg into each ramekin. Sprinkle with seasonings.
Cook for 15 minutes at 335 degrees F or until your eggs reach desired texture.
Serve warm with spicy tomato ketchup and pickles. Bon appétit!

Spicy Ground Pork Omelet with Cream Cheese

Preparation Time: 20 minutes
Servings: 2
Nutrition: 438 Calories; 22g Fat; 7g Carbs; 22g Protein; 2g Sugars; 7g Fiber
Ingredients:
4 garlic cloves, peeled and minced
1/2 tablespoon fresh basil, chopped
1/3 pound ground pork
1/3 teaspoon ground black pepper
1/2 small-sized onion, peeled and finely chopped
1 1/2 tablespoons olive oil
3 medium-sized eggs, beaten
1/2 jalapeno pepper, seeded and chopped
4 tablespoons cream cheese
1/3 teaspoon salt
Directions:
In a nonstick skillet that is preheated over a moderate flame, heat the oil; then, sweat the onion, garlic and ground pork in the hot oil.
Spritz an Air Fryer baking dish with a cooking spray.
Throw in the sautéed mixture, followed by the remaining **Ingredients:**.
Bake at 325 degrees F approximately 15 minutes. Serve with the salad of choice. Bon appétit!

Pork Belly with Lime Aromatics

Preparation Time: 1 hour 15 minutes + marinating time
Servings: 4
Nutrition: 590 Calories; 61g Fat; 5g Carbs; 16g Protein; 1g Sugars; 5g Fiber
Ingredients:
1 pound pork belly
2 garlic cloves, halved
1 teaspoon shallot powder
1 teaspoon sea salt

1 teaspoon dried basil
1 teaspoon dried oregano
1 teaspoon dried thyme
1 teaspoon dried marjoram
1 teaspoon ground black pepper
1 lime, juiced

Directions:

Blanch the pork belly in a pot of boiling water for 10 to 13 minutes.
Pat it dry with a kitchen towel. Now, poke holes all over the skin by using a fork.
Then, mix the remaining **Ingredients:** to make the rub. Massage the rub all over the pork belly.
Drizzle lime juice all over the meat; place the pork belly in the refrigerator for 3 hours.
Preheat your Air Fryer to 320 degrees F. Cook the pork belly for 35 minutes.
Turn up the temperature to 360 degrees F and continue cooking for 20 minutes longer. Serve warm. Bon appétit!

Mexican Stuffed Peppers with Pork and Cheese

Preparation Time: 30 minutes
Servings: 3
Nutrition: 425 Calories; 29g Fat; 5g Carbs; 33g Protein; 2g Sugars; 2g Fiber

Ingredients:

3 bell peppers, stems and seeds removed
1 tablespoon canola oil
1/2 cup onions, chopped
1 teaspoon fresh garlic, minced
1 Mexican chili pepper, finely chopped
1 pound lean pork, ground
1/2 teaspoon sea salt
1/2 teaspoon black pepper
1 tablespoon Mexican oregano
1 ripe tomato, pureed
3 ounces Cotija cheese, grated

Directions:

Cook the peppers in boiling salted water for 4 minutes
In a nonstick skillet, heat the canola oil over medium heat. Then, sauté the onions, garlic and Mexican chili pepper until tender and fragrant.
Stir in the ground pork and continue sautéing until the pork has browned; drain off the excess fat.
Add the salt, black pepper, Mexican oregano, and pureed tomato; give it a good stir.
Divide the filling among the bell peppers. Arrange the peppers in a baking dish lightly greased with cooking oil.
Bake in the preheated Air Fryer at 380 degrees F for 13 minutes. Top with grated Cotija cheese and bake another 6 minutes. Serve warm and enjoy!

Italian Twisted Pork Chops

Preparation Time: 20 minutes
Servings: 3
Nutrition: 517 Calories; 13g Fat; 3g Carbs; 62g Protein; 5g Sugars; 2g Fiber

Ingredients:

1/4 cup balsamic vinegar
3 center-cut loin pork chops
1/4 cup almond meal

2 tablespoons golden flaxseed meal
1 teaspoon turmeric powder
1 egg
1 teaspoon mustard
Kosher salt, to taste
1/4 teaspoon freshly ground black pepper
1/2 cup pork rinds, crushed
1/2 teaspoon garlic powder
1 teaspoon shallot powder

Directions:

Drizzle the balsamic vinegar over pork chops and spread to evenly coat.

Place the almond meal, flaxseed meal, and turmeric in a shallow bowl. In another bowl, whisk the eggs, mustard, salt, and black pepper.

In the third bowl, mix the pork rinds with the garlic powder and shallot powder.

Preheat your Air Fryer to 390 degrees F. Dredge the pork chops in the almond meal mixture, then in the egg, followed by the pork rind mixture.

Cook the pork chops for 7 minutes per side, spraying with cooking oil. Bon appétit!

Herby Pork with Celery Chips

Preparation Time: 1 hour 15 minutes
Servings: 4
Nutrition: 442 Calories; 28g Fat; 5g Carbs; 44g Protein; 2g Sugars; 3g Fiber

Ingredients:

1 tablespoon peanut oil
1 ½ pounds pork loin, cut into 4 pieces
Coarse sea salt and ground black pepper, to taste
1/2 teaspoon onion powder
1 teaspoon garlic powder
1/2 teaspoon cayenne pepper
1/2 teaspoon dried rosemary
1/2 teaspoon dried basil
1/2 teaspoon dried oregano
1 pound celery, cut into matchsticks
1 tablespoon coconut oil, melted

Directions:

Drizzle 1 tablespoon of peanut oil all over the pork loin. Season with salt, black pepper, onion powder, garlic powder, cayenne pepper, rosemary, basil, and oregano.

Cook in the preheated Air Fryer at 360 degrees F for 55 minutes; make sure to turn the pork over every 15 minutes to ensure even cooking.

Test for doneness with a meat thermometer.

Toss the carrots with melted coconut oil; season to taste and cook in the preheated Air Fryer at 380 degrees F for 15 minutes.

Serve the warm pork loin with the carrots on the side. Enjoy!

Favorite Taco Casserole

Preparation Time: 45 minutes
Servings: 4
Nutrition: 601 Calories; 49g Fat; 2g Carbs; 35g Protein; 3g Sugars; 1g Fiber

Ingredients:

1 tablespoon olive oil
1 pound pork, ground

1 tablespoon taco seasoning mix
Sea salt and ground black pepper, to taste
1 medium-sized leek, sliced
1 teaspoon fresh garlic, minced
1/2 cup celery, trimmed and sliced
1 (2-ouncejar pimiento, drained and chopped
1 can (10 ¾-ouncescondensed cream of mushroom soup
1 cup water
1/2 cup Mexican beer
1/2 cup cream cheese, grated
1 cup Mexican cheese, shredded
1 tablespoon fresh cilantro, chopped

Directions:

Start by preheating your Air Fryer to 320 degrees F.

Add the olive oil to a baking dish and heat for 1 to 2 minutes. Add the pork, taco seasoning mix, salt, pepper and cook for 6 minutes, crumbling with a fork.

Add the leeks and cook for 4 to 5 minutes, stirring occasionally.

Add the garlic, celery, pimiento, mushroom soup, water, beer, and cream cheese. Gently stir to combine.

Turn the temperature to 370 degrees F.

Top with Mexican cheese. Place the baking dish in the cooking basket and cook approximately 30 minutes or until everything is thoroughly cooked.

Serve garnished with fresh cilantro. Bon appétit!

Chinese-Style Pork Shoulder

Preparation Time: 25 minutes + marinating time
Servings: 3
Nutrition: 353 Calories; 16g Fat; 15g Carbs; 22g Protein; 12g Sugars; 2g Fiber

Ingredients:

2 tablespoons coconut aminos
2 tablespoons Shaoxing wine
2 garlic cloves, minced
1 teaspoon fresh ginger, minced
1 tablespoon cilantro stems and leaves, finely chopped
1 pound boneless pork shoulder
2 tablespoons sesame oil

Directions:

In a large-sized ceramic dish, thoroughly combine the coconut aminos, Shaoxing wine, garlic, ginger, and cilantro; add the pork shoulder and allow it to marinate for 2 hours in the refrigerator.

Then, grease the cooking basket with sesame oil. Place the pork shoulder in the cooking basket; reserve the marinade.

Cook in the preheated Air Fryer at 395 degrees F for 14 to 17 minutes, flipping and basting with the marinade halfway through. Let it rest for 5 to 6 minutes before slicing and serving.

While the pork is roasting, cook the marinade in a preheated skillet over medium heat; cook until it has thickened.

Brush the pork shoulder with the sauce and enjoy!

Cheesy Mini Meatloaves

Preparation Time: 50 minutes
Servings: 4
Nutrition: 535 Calories; 34g Fat; 8g Carbs; 41g Protein; 1g Sugars; 2g Fiber
Ingredients:
1 pound ground pork
1/2 pound ground beef
1 package onion soup mix
1/2 cup Romano cheese, grated
2 eggs
1 bell pepper, chopped
1 serrano pepper, minced
2 scallions, chopped
2 cloves garlic, finely chopped
Sea salt and black pepper, to your liking
Glaze:
1/2 cup tomato paste
1 tablespoon brown mustard
1 teaspoon smoked paprika
Directions:
In a large mixing bowl, thoroughly combine all **Ingredients:** for meatloaves. Mix with your hands until everything is well incorporated.
Then, shape the mixture into four mini loaves. Transfer them to the cooking basket previously generously greased with cooking oil.
Cook in the preheated Air Fryer at 385 degrees F approximately 43 minutes.
Mix all **Ingredients:** for the glaze. Spread the glaze over mini meatloaves and cook for another 6 minutes. Bon appétit!

Bacon Cheese-burger Casserole

Preparation Time: 35 minutes
Servings: 4
Ingredients:
1 lb. 80/20 ground beef.
4 slices sugar-free bacon; cooked and crumbled
1 large egg.
2 pickle spears; chopped
¼ medium white onion; peeled. And chopped
1 cup shredded Cheddar cheese, divided.
Directions:
Brown the ground beef in a medium skillet over medium heat about 7–10 minutes. When no pink remains, drain the fat. Remove from heat and add ground beef to large mixing bowl.
Add onion, ½ cup Cheddar and egg to bowl. Mix **Ingredients:** well and add crumbled bacon
Pour the mixture into a 4-cup round baking dish and top with remaining Cheddar. Place into the air fryer basket. Adjust the temperature to 375 Degrees F and set the timer for 20 minutes
Casserole will be golden on top and firm in the middle when fully cooked. Serve immediately with chopped pickles on top.
Nutrition: Calories: 369; Protein: 30g; Fiber: 2g; Fat: 26g; Carbs: 2g

Pork with Lemon Sauce

Preparation Time: 40 minutes
Servings: 4
Ingredients:
4 pork chops
2 garlic cloves; minced
2 tbsp. olive oil
4 tsp. mustard
2 tsp. lemon zest, grated
Juice of 1 lemon
A pinch of salt and black pepper
Directions:
Take a bowl and mix the pork chops with the other **Ingredients:**, toss and keep in the fridge for 15 minutes
Put the pork chops in your air fryer's basket and cook at 390°F for 25 minutes. Divide between plates and serve with a side salad.
Nutrition: Calories: 287; Fat: 13g; Fiber: 4g; Carbs: 6g; Protein: 20g

Chipotle Pork Chops

Preparation Time: 40 minutes
Servings: 4
Ingredients:
4 pork chops, bone-in
2 ½ tbsp. ghee; melted
½ tsp. allspice
1 tsp. coconut sugar
½ tsp. garlic powder
½ tsp. chipotle chili powder
½ tsp. cinnamon powder
A pinch of salt and black pepper
Directions:
Rub the pork chops with all the other **Ingredients:**, put them in your air fryer's basket and cook at 380°F for 35 minutes
Divide the chops between plates and serve with a side salad.
Nutrition: Calories: 287; Fat: 14g; Fiber: 4g; Carbs: 7g; Protein: 18g

Mustard Pork Chops

Preparation Time: 30 minutes
Servings: 4
Ingredients:
4 pork chops
10 oz. beef stock
2/3 cup cream cheese, soft
1 tbsp. olive oil
1 tbsp. mustard
1 tbsp. parsley; chopped
¼ tsp. oregano; dried
¼ tsp. thyme; dried
¼ tsp. garlic powder
A pinch of salt and black pepper

Directions:
In a baking dish that fits your air fryer, mix all the Ingredients:, introduce the pan in the fryer and cook at 400°F for 25 minutes
Divide everything between plates and serve.
Nutrition: Calories: 284; Fat: 14g; Fiber: 4g; Carbs: 6g; Protein: 22

Lamb Meatloaf

Preparation Time: 40 minutes
Servings: 4
Ingredients:
2 lb. lamb, ground
4 scallions; chopped
1 egg
A drizzle of olive oil
2 tbsp. tomato sauce
2 tbsp. parsley; chopped
2 tbsp. cilantro; chopped
¼ tsp. cinnamon powder
1 tsp. coriander, ground
1 tsp. lemon juice
½ tsp. hot paprika
1 tsp. cumin, ground
A pinch of salt and black pepper
Directions:
In a bowl, combine the lamb with the rest of the **Ingredients:** except the oil and stir really well.
Grease a loaf pan that fits the air fryer with the oil, add the lamb mix and shape the meatloaf
Put the pan in the air fryer and cook at 380°F for 35 minutes. Slice and serve
Nutrition: Calories: 263; Fat: 12g; Fiber: 3g; Carbs: 6g; Protein: 15g

Chives and Mustard Beef

Preparation Time: 25 minutes
Servings: 4
Ingredients:
1 ½ lb. beef; cut into strips
3 garlic cloves; minced
2 cups baby spinach
4 tbsp. mustard
2 tbsp. coconut oil; melted
2 tbsp. chives; chopped
Salt and black pepper to taste.
Directions:
In a pan that fits the air fryer, combine all the **Ingredients:**.
Put the pan in the air fryer and cook at 390°F for 20 minutes. Divide between plates and serve
Nutrition: Calories: 283; Fat: 14g; Fiber: 2g; Carbs: 6g; Protein: 19g

Easy Pork Chops

Preparation Time: 25 minutes
Servings: 4
Ingredients:
1½ oz. pork rinds, finely ground
1 tsp. chili powder

½ tsp. garlic powder.
1 tbsp. coconut oil; melted
4 (4-oz.pork chops

Directions:

Take a large bowl, mix ground pork rinds, chili powder and garlic powder.
Brush each pork chop with coconut oil and then press into the pork rind mixture, coating both sides. Place each coated pork chop into the air fryer basket
Adjust the temperature to 400 Degrees F and set the timer for 15 minutes. Flip each pork chop halfway through the cooking time
When fully cooked the pork chops will be golden on the outside and have an internal temperature of at least 145 Degrees F.

Nutrition: Calories: 292; Protein: 25g; Fiber: 3g; Fat: 15g; Carbs: 6g

Coconut and Chili Pork

Preparation Time: 30 minutes
Servings: 4
Ingredients:

4 pork chops
2 garlic cloves; minced
1 shallot; chopped
1 ½ cups coconut milk
3 tbsp. coconut aminos
2 tbsp. olive oil
2 tsp. chili paste
Salt and black pepper to taste.

Directions:

In a pan that fits your air fryer, mix the pork the rest of the **Ingredients:**, toss, introduce the pan in the fryer and cook at 400°F for 25 minutes, shaking the fryer halfway.
Divide everything into bowls and serve.

Nutrition: Calories: 267; Fat: 12g; Fiber: 4g; Carbs: 6g; Protein: 18g

BBQ Meatballs

Preparation Time: 24 minutes
Servings: 4
Ingredients:

¼ lb. ground Italian sausage
1 lb. 80/20 ground beef.
4 slices sugar-free bacon; cooked and chopped
¼ cup chopped white onion
¼ cup chopped pickled jalapeños.
½ cup low-carb, sugar-free barbecue sauce
1 large egg.
1 tsp. dried parsley.
¼ tsp. onion powder.
½ tsp. garlic powder.

Directions:

Take a large bowl, mix ground beef, sausage and egg until fully combined. Mix in all remaining **Ingredients:** except barbecue sauce. Form into eight meatballs. Place meatballs into the air fryer basket.
Adjust the temperature to 400 Degrees F and set the timer for 14 minutes
Turn the meatballs halfway through the cooking time

When done, meatballs should be browned on the outside and have an internal temperature of at least 180 Degrees F. Remove meatballs from fryer and toss in barbecue sauce. Serve warm.
Nutrition: Calories: 336; Protein: 21g; Fiber: 4g; Fat: 15g; Carbs: 4g

Pork Roast

Preparation Time: 35 minutes
Servings: 4
Ingredients:
1 lb. pork tenderloin, trimmed
2 tbsp. balsamic vinegar
3 tbsp. mustard
2 tbsp. olive oil
A pinch of salt and black pepper
Directions:
Take a bowl and mix the pork tenderloin with the rest of the **Ingredients:** and rub well.
Put the roast in your air fryer's basket and cook at 380°F for 30 minutes. Slice the roast, divide between plates and serve.
Nutrition: Calories: 274; Fat: 13g; Fiber: 4g; Carbs: 7g; Protein: 22

Seared Ribeye

Preparation Time: 50 minutes
Servings: 2
Ingredients:
1 (8-oz.ribeye steak
1 tbsp. salted butter; softened.
1 tbsp. coconut oil
½ tsp. dried parsley.
½ tsp. pink Himalayan salt
¼ tsp. ground peppercorn
¼ tsp. dried oregano.
¼ tsp. garlic powder.
Directions:
Rub steak with salt and ground peppercorn. Place into the air fryer basket.
Adjust the temperature to 250 Degrees F and set the timer for 45 minutes.
After timer beeps, begin checking doneness and add a few minutes until internal temperature is your personal preference
In a medium skillet over medium heat, add coconut oil. When oil is hot, quickly sear outside and sides of steak until crisp and browned. Remove from heat and allow steak to rest
In a small bowl, whip butter with garlic powder, parsley and oregano. Slice steak and serve with herb butter on top.
Nutrition: Calories: 377; Protein: 26g; Fiber: 2g; Fat: 37g; Carbs: 6g

Fajita Flank Steak Rolls

Preparation Time: 35 minutes
Servings: 6
Ingredients:
2 lb. flank steak
4 (1-oz.slices pepper jack cheese
1 medium red bell pepper; seeded and sliced into strips
¼ cup diced yellow onion
1 medium green bell pepper; seeded and sliced into strips

2 tbsp. unsalted butter.
1 tsp. cumin
½ tsp. garlic powder.
2 tsp. chili powder

Directions:

In a medium skillet over medium heat, melt butter and begin sautéing onion, red bell pepper and green bell pepper. Sprinkle with chili powder, cumin and garlic powder. Sauté until peppers are tender, about 5–7 minutes.
Lay flank steak flat on a work surface. Spread onion and pepper mixture over entire steak rectangle. Lay slices of cheese on top of onions and peppers, barely overlapping
With the shortest end toward you, begin rolling the steak, tucking the cheese down into the roll as necessary.
Secure the roll with twelve toothpicks, six on each side of the steak roll. Place steak roll into the air fryer basket
Adjust the temperature to 400 Degrees F and set the timer for 15 minutes. Rotate the roll halfway through the cooking time. Add an additional 1–4 minutes depending on your preferred internal temperature (135 Degrees F for medium
When timer beeps, allow roll to rest 15 minutes, then slice into six even pieces. Serve warm.
Nutrition: Calories: 439; Protein: 30g; Fiber: 2g; Fat: 26g; Carbs: 7g

Lamb Chops and Mint Sauce

Preparation Time: 29 minutes
Servings: 4
Ingredients:

8 lamb chops
1 cup mint; chopped
1 garlic clove; minced
2 tbsp. olive oil
Juice of 1 lemon
A pinch of salt and black pepper

Directions:

In a blender, combine all the **Ingredients:** except the lamb and pulse well.
Rub lamb chops with the mint sauce, put them in your air fryer's basket and cook at 400°F for 12 minutes on each side
Divide everything between plates and serve.
Nutrition: Calories: 284; Fat: 14g; Fiber: 3g; Carbs: 6g; Protein: 16g

Rosemary Roasted Lamb Cutlets

Preparation Time: 35 minutes
Servings: 4
Ingredients:

8 lamb cutlets
2 garlic cloves; minced
2 tbsp. rosemary; chopped
2 tbsp. olive oil
A pinch of salt and black pepper
A pinch of cayenne pepper

Directions:

Take a bowl and mix the lamb with the rest of the **Ingredients:** and rub well.
Put the lamb in the fryer's basket and cook at 380°F for 30 minutes, flipping them halfway.
Divide the cutlets between plates and serve

Nutrition: Calories: 274; Fat: 12g; Fiber: 3g; Carbs: 5g; Protein: 15g

Seasoned Lamb

Preparation Time: 40 minutes
Servings: 4
Ingredients:
1 lb. lamb leg; boneless and sliced
½ cup walnuts; chopped
2 garlic cloves; minced
1 tbsp. parsley; chopped
1 tbsp. rosemary; chopped
2 tbsp. olive oil
¼ tsp. red pepper flakes
½ tsp. mustard seeds
½ tsp. Italian seasoning
A pinch of salt and black pepper
Directions:
Take a bowl and mix the lamb with all the **Ingredients:** except the walnuts and parsley, rub well, put the slices your air fryer's basket and cook at 370°F for 35 minutes, flipping the meat halfway
Divide between plates, sprinkle the parsley and walnuts on top and serve with a side salad
Nutrition: Calories: 283; Fat: 13g; Fiber: 4g; Carbs: 6g; Protein: 15g

Herbed Lamb

Preparation Time: 40 minutes
Servings: 4
Ingredients:
8 lamb cutlets
¼ cup mustard
2 garlic cloves; minced
1 tbsp. oregano; chopped
1 tbsp. mint chopped.
1 tbsp. chives; chopped
1 tbsp. basil; chopped
A drizzle of olive oil
A pinch of salt and black pepper
Directions:
Take a bowl and mix the lamb with the rest of the **Ingredients:** and rub well.
Put the cutlets in your air fryer's basket and cook at 380°F for 15 minutes on each side
Divide between plates and serve with a side salad.
Nutrition: Calories: 284; Fat: 13g; Fiber: 3g; Carbs: 6g; Protein: 14g

Smoked Pork Chops

Preparation Time: 30 minutes
Servings: 4
Ingredients:
4 pork chops
½ cup chicken stock
2 tbsp. balsamic vinegar
1 tbsp. smoked paprika
1 tbsp. olive oil

A pinch of salt and black pepper

Directions:

Take a bowl and mix the pork chops with the rest of the **Ingredients:** and toss.

Put the pork chops in your air fryer's basket and cook at 390°F for 25 minutes

Divide between plates and serve.

Nutrition: Calories: 276; Fat: 12g; Fiber: 4g; Carbs: 6g; Protein: 22

Bacon Wrapped Hot Dog.

Preparation Time: 15 minutes

Servings: 4

Ingredients:

4 slices sugar-free bacon.

4 beef hot dogs

Directions:

Wrap each hot dog with slice of bacon and secure with toothpick. Place into the air fryer basket. Adjust the temperature to 370 Degrees F and set the timer for 10 minutes. Flip each hot dog halfway through the cooking time. When fully cooked, bacon will be crispy. Serve warm.

Nutrition: Calories: 197; Protein: 2g; Fiber: 0g; Fat: 10g; Carbs: 3g

Beef and Balsamic Marinade

Preparation Time: 40 minutes

Servings: 4

Ingredients:

4 medium beef steaks

3 garlic cloves; minced

1 cup balsamic vinegar

2 tbsp. olive oil

Salt and black pepper to taste.

Directions:

Take a bowl and mix steaks with the rest of the **Ingredients:** and toss.

Transfer the steaks to your air fryer's basket and cook at 390°F for 35 minutes, flipping them halfway

Divide between plates and serve with a side salad.

Nutrition: Calories: 273; Fat: 14g; Fiber: 4g; Carbs: 6g; Protein: 19g

Pub Burger

Preparation Time: 20 minutes

Servings: 4

Ingredients:

8 large leaves butter lettuce

1 lb. ground sirloin

4 Bacon-Wrapped Onion Rings

½ cup full-fat mayonnaise

8 slices pickle

2 tbsp. salted butter; melted.

2 tsp. sriracha

¼ tsp. garlic powder.

½ tsp. salt

¼ tsp. ground black pepper

Directions:

Take a medium bowl, combine ground sirloin, salt and pepper. Form four patties. Brush each with butter and then place into the air fryer basket. Adjust the temperature to 380 Degrees F and set the timer for 10 minutes

Flip the patties halfway through the cooking time for a medium burger. Add an additional 3–5 minutes for well-done

In a small bowl, mix mayonnaise, sriracha and garlic powder. Set aside.

Place each cooked burger on a lettuce leaf and top with onion ring, two pickles and dollop of your prepared burger sauce. Wrap another lettuce leaf around tightly to hold. Serve warm.

Nutrition: Calories: 442; Protein: 23g; Fiber: 8g; Fat: 39g; Carbs: 1g

Lasagna Casserole

Preparation Time: 30 minutes

Servings: 4

Ingredients:

¾ cup low-carb no-sugar-added pasta sauce

1 lb. 80/20 ground beef; cooked and drained

½ cup full-fat ricotta cheese

¼ cup grated Parmesan cheese.

½ tsp. garlic powder.

1 tsp. dried parsley.

½ tsp. dried oregano.

1 cup shredded mozzarella cheese

Directions:

In a 4-cup round baking dish, pour ¼ cup pasta sauce on the bottom of the dish. Place ¼ of the ground beef on top of the sauce.

In a small bowl, mix ricotta, Parmesan, garlic powder, parsley and oregano. Place dollops of half the mixture on top of the beef

Sprinkle with ⅓ of the mozzarella. Repeat layers until all beef, ricotta mixture, sauce and mozzarella are used, ending with the mozzarella on top

Cover dish with foil and place into the air fryer basket. Adjust the temperature to 370 Degrees F and set the timer for 15 minutes. In the last 2 minutes of cooking, remove the foil to brown the cheese. Serve immediately.

Nutrition: Calories: 371; Protein: 34g; Fiber: 6g; Fat: 24g; Carbs: 8g

Beef and Radishes

Preparation Time: 20 minutes

Servings: 2

Ingredients:

1 lb. radishes, quartered

2 cups corned beef, cooked and shredded

2 spring onions; chopped

2 garlic cloves; minced

A pinch of salt and black pepper

Directions:

In a pan that fits your air fryer, mix the beef with the rest of the Ingredients:, toss.

Put the pan in the fryer and cook at 390°F for 15 minutes

Divide everything into bowls and serve.

Nutrition: Calories: 267; Fat: 13g; Fiber: 2g; Carbs: 5g; Protein: 15g

Spicy Beef

Preparation Time: 25 minutes
Servings: 4
Ingredients:
4 beef steaks
1 tbsp. hot paprika
1 tbsp. butter; melted
Salt and black pepper to taste.
Directions:
Take a bowl and mix the beef with the rest of the **Ingredients:**, rub well, transfer the steaks to your air fryer's basket and cook at 390°F for 10 minutes on each side
Divide the steaks between plates and serve with a side salad.
Nutrition: Calories: 280; Fat: 12g; Fiber: 4g; Carbs: 6g; Protein: 17g

Adobo Beef

Preparation Time: 35 minutes
Servings: 4
Ingredients:
1 lb. beef roast, trimmed
1 tbsp. olive oil
¼ tsp. garlic powder
½ tsp. turmeric powder
½ tsp. oregano; dried
A pinch of salt and black pepper
Directions:
Take a bowl and mix the roast with the rest of the **Ingredients:** and rub well.
Put the roast in the air fryer's basket and cook at 390°F for 30 minutes. Slice the roast, divide it between plates and serve with a side salad.
Nutrition: Calories: 294; Fat: 12g; Fiber: 3g; Carbs: 6g; Protein: 19g

Steak

Preparation Time: 10 minutes
Cooking time: 15 minutes

Servings: 1 to 3 people
Recipe **Ingredients:**
2 strip loin steaks (25" thick
2 teaspoons of salt (plus more to taste
2 teaspoons of black pepper (plus more to taste
2 tablespoons of butter (melted
Direction:
Sprinkle the steaks with salt and pepper.
place on a plate and refrigerate for about 2 to 3 days, uncovered. Flip every 12 hours or so, blotting the juices with a paper towel.
This step is recommended for superior tenderness and enhanced flavor, but you can skip it if pressed for time.
Remove the steaks from the fridge 45 to 60 minutes before cooking and let them sit at room temperature.
Brush the steaks with melted butter on both sides, place inside your air fryer. Cook at 4100F for about 15 minutes, without pre-heating, for medium doneness.

Cook for about 1 to 2 minutes less for medium rare and rare respectively, and 1-2 minutes more for medium-well and well done respectively.
The times will need to be adjusted further if air frying steaks thicker or thinner than 25" thick. Use an instant read thermometer to check for doneness. Remove steaks from the air fryer, wrap in foil or wax paper, and let rest for 10 minutes, then serve.

Roast Beef

Preparation Time: 5 minutes
Cooking time: 35 minutes
Overall time: 40 minutes
Servings: 2 to 4 people
Recipe **Ingredients:**
2 pounds of beef roast top round or eye of round is best
Oil for spraying
Rub
1 tablespoon of kosher salt
1 teaspoon of black pepper
2 teaspoons of garlic powder
1 teaspoon of summer savory
Direction:
Mix all rub **Ingredients:** and rub into roast. Place fat side down in the basket of the air fryer. Lightly spray with oil.
Set fryer to 4000F and air fry for about 20 minutes; turn fat-side up and spray lightly with oil. Continue cooking for 15 additional minutes at 4000F. Remove the roast from the fryer, tent with foil and let the meat rest for 10 minutes.
The time given should produce a rare roast which should be 1250F on a meat thermometer. Additional time will be needed for medium, medium-well and well.
Always use a meat thermometer to test the temperature. Approximate times for medium and well respectively are 40 minutes and 45 minutes.
Remember to always use a meat thermometer to check for doneness. Serve immediately and Enjoy!

Steak and Asparagus Bundles

Preparation Time: 5 minutes
Cooking time: 15 minutes

Servings: 2 to 4 people
Recipe **Ingredients:**
2 (2 ½ poundsof Flank steak - cut into 6 pieces
Kosher salt/black pepper
½ cup of tamari sauce
2 cloves of garlic - crushed
1 lb. of asparagus - trimmed
3 bell peppers - seeded and sliced thinly
¼ cup of balsamic vinegar
1/3 cup of beef broth
2 tbsp. of unsalted butter
Olive oil spray
Direction:
Season steaks with salt and pepper. Place steaks into a large zip top bag. Add tamari sauce and garlic and seal the bag.

Massage steaks so that they're completely coated. Transfer to refrigerator and allow to marinade for a minimum of 1 hour up to overnight.
When ready to assemble, remove steaks from marinade and place on a cutting board or sheet. Discard marinade.
Equally divide and then place asparagus and bell peppers into the middle of each piece of steak. Roll steak around vegetables and secure with tooth picks.
Preheat air fryer. Working in batches, depending on the size of your air fryer, place bundles into basket of air fryer. Spray vegetables with olive oil spray.
Cook at 4000F for about 5 minutes. Remove steak bundles and allow to rest for 5 minutes prior to serving/slicing.
While the steak is resting, into small-medium sauce pan heat: balsamic vinegar, broth and butter over medium heat. Whisk to combine.
Continue cooking until sauce has thickened and reduced by half. Season with salt and pepper. Pour sauce over steak bundles prior to serving.

Beef & Bean Chimichangas

Preparation Time: 15 minutes
Cooking time: 8 minutes
Overall time: 23 minutes
Servings: 8 to 10 people
Recipe **Ingredients:**
1 lb. of ground beef
1 package of taco seasoning
½ cup of refried beans
½ cup of shredded colby jack cheese
10 taco size flour tortillas or 5 burrito flour size tortillas
Toppings:
Queso
Lettuce
Tomato
Sour cream
Salsa
Direction:
Brown the ground beef and add the taco seasoning as instructed. Once the meat is cooked, mix in the refried beans.
Add the mixture to the middle of each tortillas and top with shredded cheese. Fold the tortilla up to be sure that all the toppings are securely inside the tortilla.
Spray the air fryer with non-stick cooking spray or olive oil spray. Place the chimichangas seam side down into the air fryer.
Spray them with a coat of olive oil spray. This can also be done with avocado cooking spray. Cook at 3600F, for about 8 minutes.
Check on them at the 5th minutes to be sure they are cooking nicely. Once done they should be lightly browned on top and the tortilla will be nicely secured. Serve immediately and Enjoy!

Raspberry Balsamic Smoked Pork Chops

Preparation Time: 15 minutes
Cooking time: 15 minutes
Overall time: 30 minutes
Servings: 2 to 4 people
Recipe **Ingredients:**
2 large eggs

¼ cup of milk
1 cup of panko (Japanesebread crumbs
1 cup of finely chopped pecans
4 smoked bone-in pork chops (7-1/2 ounces each
¼ cup of all-purpose flour
1/3 cup of balsamic vinegar
2 tbsp. of brown sugar
2 tbsp. of seedless raspberry jam
1 tbsp. of thawed frozen orange juice concentrate
Cooking **Directions:**
Preheat air fryer to 400°F and Spritz air fryer basket with cooking spray. In a shallow bowl, whisk together eggs and milk.
In another shallow bowl, toss bread crumbs with pecans. Coat pork chops with flour; shake off excess.
Dip in egg mixture, then in crumb mixture, patting to help adhere. Working in batches as needed. Place chops in single layer in air fryer basket and spritz with cooking spray. Cook until golden brown, for about 12 to 15 minutes.
Turn halfway through cooking and spritzing with additional cooking spray. Remove and keep warm. Repeat with remaining chops.
Meanwhile, place remaining **Ingredients:** in a small saucepan; bring to a boil. Cook and stir until slightly thickened, for about 6 to 8 minutes. Serve with chops.

Mongolian Beef

Preparation Time: 20 minutes
Cooking time: 20 minutes
Overall time: 40 minutes
Servings: 2 to 4 people
Recipe **Ingredients:**
Meat:
1 pound of flank steak
¼ cup of corn starch
sauce:
2 teaspoons of vegetable oil
½ teaspoon of ginger
1 tablespoon of minced garlic
½ cup of soy sauce or gluten free soy sauce
½ cup of water
¾ cup of brown sugar, packed
extras:
Cooked rice
Green beans
Green onions
Direction:
Thinly slice the steak in long pieces, then coat with the corn starch. Place in the Air Fryer and cook on 390* for 5 minutes on each side.
While the steak cooks, warm up all sauce ingredient in a medium sized saucepan on medium-high heat. Whisk the **Ingredients:** together until it gets to a low boil.
Once both the steak and sauce are cooked, place the steak in a bowl with the sauce and let it soak in for about 5 to 10 minutes.
When ready to serve, use tongs to remove the steak and let the excess sauce drip off.
Place steak on cooked rice and green beans, top with additional sauce if you prefer.

Pork Chops

Preparation Time: 5 minutes
Cooking time: 16 minutes
Overall time: 21 minutes
Servings: 2 to 4 people
Recipe **Ingredients:**
4 boneless pork chops
½ tsp. of salt
¼ tsp. of sugar
½ tsp. of granulated garlic
½ tsp. of granulated onion
½ tsp. of parsley
½ tsp. of celery seed
2 tsp. of oil
Direction:
Mix together the seasonings and then sprinkle onto both sides of the pork chops.
After seasoning put the oil on the pork chops and rub it in. You could also use spray oil.
Cook the pork chops at 3500F, for about 5 minutes per side for thin and 8 minutes per side for thick.
The pork chops are done when they reach 145° F measured in the center, this is the lowest safe point for pork chops. Go to about 155 to 1600F for well-done pork chops.
Serve immediately and Enjoy!

Char Siu Pork

Preparation Time: 10 minutes
Cooking time: 20 minutes
Overall time: 30 minutes
Servings: 2 to 4 people
Recipe **Ingredients:**
4 tbsp. of honey
2 tbsp. of dark soy sauce
1 tbsp. of sugar
1 tbsp. of Shaoxing (rice cooking wine
1 tbsp. of hoisin sauce
2 tsp. of minced garlic
2 tsp. of minced ginger
1 tsp. of Chinese five spice
1 lb. boneless pork shoulder or pork belly
Direction:
Using a fork, pierce the slices of pork well. Mix all **Ingredients:** for the sauce (except the pork shouldertogether in a small microwave-safe bowl.
Place the pork slices in a zip lock bag or bowl, and pour in half the sauce. Mix well and let the pork marinate for 30 minutes, and up to 24 hours in the refrigerator.
Remove pork from the marinade and place in a single layer in your air fryer basket. Set the air fryer to 3900F for about 15 minutes, flipping the pork half way through.
While the Char Siu is cooking, place the reserved half of the sauce in the microwave and cook on high for about 45 to 60 seconds stirring every 15 seconds.
You are doing this to thicken the sauce a little. Since it has honey in it, be careful to not overcook otherwise you will have char siu toffee.

Using a meat thermometer, ensure your pork has reached an internal temperature of 1450F.Remove the pork to a cutting board and let it rest for 10 minutes.
Brush with the thickened, cooked sauce and serve.

Crispy Pork Belly

Preparation Time: 10 minutes
Cooking time: 30 minutes

Servings: 2 to 5 people
Recipe **Ingredients:**
1 lb. of pork belly
3 cups of water
1 tsp. of salt
1 tsp. of ground black pepper
2 tbsp. of soy sauce
2 bay leaves
6 cloves of garlic
Direction:
Cut the pork belly into 3 thick chunks so that it cooks more evenly. Place all **Ingredients:** into the inner liner of an Instant Pot or pressure cooker.
Cook the pork belly at high pressure for about 15 minutes. Allow the pot to sit undisturbed for 10 minutes and then release all remaining pressure.
Using a set of tongs, very carefully remove the meat from the pressure cooker. Allow the meat to drain and dry for 10 minutes.
If you do not have a pressure cooker, place the **Ingredients:** into a sauce pan, cover, and cook for about 60 minutes, until a knife can be easily inserted into the skin-side of the pork belly.
Remove the meat and allow the meat to drain and dry for 10 minutes. Cut each of the three chunks of pork belly into 2 long slices.
Place the pork belly slices in the air fryer basket. Set the air fryer to 400°F for about 15 minutes or until the fat on the pork belly has crisped up, and then serve.

Beef kabobs

Preparation Time: 30 minutes
Cooking time: 10 minutes
Overall time: 40 minutes
Servings: 2 to 4 people
Recipe **Ingredients:**
1 pound of beef chuck ribs cut in 1 inch pieces
1/3 cup of low fat sour cream
2 tablespoons of soy sauce
8 (6 inchof skewers
1 bell peppers
½ onion
Direction:
Mix sour cream with soy sauce in a medium bowl. Place beef chunks into the bowl and marinate for at least 30 minuteso better overnight.
Cut bell pepper and onion in 1 inch pieces. Soak wooden skewers in water for about 10 minutes.
Thread beef, onions and bell peppers onto skewers. Add some freshly ground black pepper.
Cook in preheated to 4000F Air fryer for about 10 minutes, turning half way. Serve immediately and Enjoy!

Rack of Lamb

Preparation Time: 5 minutes
Cooking time: 10 minutes

Servings: 2 to 4 people
Recipe **Ingredients:**
1 rack of lamb
2 tbsp. of dried rosemary
1 tbsp. of dried thyme
2 tsp. of minced garlic
Salt
Pepper
4 tbsp. of olive oil
Direction:
Start by making your mixture of herbs, mix in a small bowl, the rosemary, thyme, garlic, salt, pepper, and olive oil and combine well.
Then rub the mixture all over the lamb. Place the rack of lamb into the air fryer. Set the temperature to 3600F, for about 10 minutes.
After 10 minutes, measure your internal temperature of the rack of lamb by using the method above. If you want rare it would be 1450F.
If you want medium it would be 1600F. If you want well done, it would be 1700 F. Then remove, plate and serve.

Lamb Sirloin Steak

Preparation Time: 40 minutes
Cooking time: 15 minutes
Overall time:55 minutes
Servings: 2 to 4 people
Recipe **Ingredients:**
½ onion
4 slices of ginger
5 cloves of garlic
1 tsp of garam masala
1 tsp. of ground fennel
1 tsp. of ground cinnamon
½ tsp. of ground cardamom
1 tsp. of cayenne
1 tsp. of salt
1 lb. of boneless lamb sirloin steaks
Direction:
Into a blender bowl, add all **Ingredients:** except the lamb chops.
Pulse and blend until the onion is minced fine and all **Ingredients:** are blended, for about 3 to 4 minutes.
Place the lamb chops into a large bowl. Use a knife to slash into the meat and fat to allow the marinade to penetrate better.
Add the blended spice paste and mix well. Allow the mixture to rest for 30 minutes or up to 24 hours in a refrigerator.
Let your air fryer to 3300F for about 15 minutes and place the lamb steaks in a single layer in the air fryer basket and cook, flipping half way through.

Using a meat thermometer, ensure that the meat has reached an internal temperature of 150F for medium well, and serve.

Beef Jerky

Preparation Time: 5 minutes
Cooking time: 30 minutes
Ingredients:
1 pound of bottom round beef, sliced into thin strips
½ cup of dark brown sugar
½ cup of soy sauce
¼ cup of Worcestershire sauce
1 tablespoon of hickory liquid smoke
1 tablespoon chili pepper sauce
1 teaspoon of onion powder
1 teaspoon of garlic powder
1 teaspoon of cayenne red pepper
½ teaspoon of smoked paprika
½ teaspoon of ground pepper
Direction:
Prepare your **Ingredients:**. Mix all of the **Ingredients:** except for the meat in a bowl. This will create your marinade.
Slice your beef thinly but if it's still too thick, you can use a mallet to reduce its thickness. Place the meat slices inside the marinade bowl.
Make sure that each slide is well coated so your jerky can really absorb the flavor of your marinade. Cover the bowl and let it sit overnight.
Pre-heat the air fryer to 1800F. Then pat dry the marinated beef strips with paper towels. There are two ways you can go about air frying beef jerky.
You can try both to discover the best way to get the job done. Use barbecue sticks to cook them on a skewer.
You'll basically hang the strips of meat using a stick so it can be better exposed to the hot air inside the air fryer.
Puncture one end of the strips and then place the sticks across the fry basket to achieve this.
Layer the meat. You can use a cooking rack for this method. Lay out some of the marinated strips in the bottom of the fry basket then place a cooking rack on top.
Lay out another batch of marinated beef strips on top of that. Set the air fryer to 1800F then cook for an hour. Enjoy!

Beef Satay

Preparation Time: 5 minutes
Cooking time: 30 minutes
Overall time: 35 minutes
Servings: 8 to 10 people
Recipe **Ingredients:**
2 tbsp. of soy sauce
1 tsp. of sesame oil
1 tsp. of minced fresh ginger
1 tsp. of minced garlic
½ tsp. of chili garlic sauce, or more to taste
1 ¼ lb. of strip steak, rib-eye or filet, sliced into long thin strips
Peanut Sauce:
1 tbsp. of chopped green onions

1 tbsp. of chopped cilantro
1 tbsp. of minced jalapeno
½ tsp. of minced garlic
¼ tsp. of minced ginger
½ cup of coconut milk
1/3 cup of smooth peanut butter
1 tbsp. of fish sauce
1 tbsp. of lime juice
1 tbsp. of hoisin sauce
Chopped roasted peanuts, for garnish
Cilantro leaves, for garnish
Sticky rice, for serving
Lettuce leaves, for serving
Direction:
To make the beef satay, combine the soy sauce, sesame oil, ginger, garlic and chili garlic sauce and stir well. Add the beef to the sauce and toss to coat.
Marinate for 1 hour in the refrigerator. Remove the beef from the marinade and thread one strip of beef on a soaked wooden bamboo skewer.
Place on a baking sheet and continue with the remaining beef and skewers. Transfer 4 or 5 skewers to the basket of the Emeril Air Fryer set to 370° F.
When the timer goes off transfer the first batch of skewers to a platter and cover until ready to serve. Repeat with the remaining beef and skewers.
Prepare the Peanut sauce. In a food processor, combine the green onions, cilantro, jalapeno, garlic and ginger and process on high speed for 30 seconds.
Transfer the vegetables to a small mixing bowl and set aside. Add the coconut milk, peanut butter, fish sauce, lime juice and hoisin sauce to the food processor and blend until smooth.
Transfer the peanut butter mixture to the bowl with the vegetables and stir until well combined.
The peanut sauce can be made up to 3 days in advance and stored in the refrigerator for up to 1 week.
Serve the Beef Satay with the Peanut Sauce, sticky rice, lettuce leaves, chopped roasted peanuts and cilantro leaves.

Paleo Sirloin Steak

Preparation Time: 10 minutes
Cooking time: 10 minutes
Overall time: 20 minutes
Servings: 2 to 4 people
Recipe **Ingredients:**
2 Sirloin Steaks
2 tablespoons of Primal Palate Steak Seasoning
Cooking Fat (ghee, coconut oil or avocado oil
Direction:
Preheat your air fryer for about 5 minutes at 3920F. Remove the steak from the fridge and pat dry.
Brush (or spraythe top of the sirloin with cooking fat (about 1-2 tsp.and season generously.
Coat the bottom of the air fryer basket in cooking fat and add the sirloin steak to the basket. Cook for about 5 minutes.
Flip the sirloin steak and cook an additional 5 minutes. Remove the steak from the air fryer and let it rest for 5 minutes before slicing and servings.

Lasagna

Preparation Time: 5 minutes
Cooking time:
Ingredients:
For the meat layer:
Extra-virgin olive oil
1 lb. of 85% lean ground beef
1 cup of prepared marinara sauce
¼ cup of diced celery
¼ cup of diced red onion
½ tsp. of minced garlic
Salt and pepper
For the cheese layer:
8 oz. of ricotta cheese
1 cup of shredded cheese, divided
½ cup of grated parmesan cheese
2 large eggs
1 tsp. of dried Italian seasoning
½ tsp. of minced garlic
Direction:
For the meat layer: Grease a 5-inch barrel cake pan with 1 teaspoon olive oil.
In a large bowl, combine the ground beef, marinara, celery, onion, garlic, salt, and pepper. Place the seasoned meat in the pan.
Place the pan in the air fryer basket, set the air to 375F for 10 minutes. In a medium bowl, combine the ricotta, half the mozzarella, parmesan, lightly beaten eggs, Italian seasoning, and minced garlic.
Stir until well blended. At the end of the cooking time, spread the cheese mixture over the meat mixture.
Sprinkle with the remaining ½ cup mozzarella. Set the air fryer to 3750F for 10 minutes, or until the cheese is browned and bubbling.
At the end of the cooking time, use a meat thermometer to ensure the meat has reached an internal temperature of 1600F.
Drain the fat and liquid form the pan. Let stand for 5 minutes before serving.

Roast lamb

Preparation Time: 5 minutes
Cooking time: 90 minutes

Servings: 2 to 5 people
Recipe **Ingredients:**
25kg half lamb leg roast
2 cloves of garlic sliced into smaller slithers
1 tablespoon of dried rosemary
2 tablespoons of olive oil (optional
Cracked Himalayan rock salt and cracked peppercorns
Direction:
Make deep slits in the lamb fat on top using the point of a knife. Poke garlic slithers into the slits.
Rub or brush on mix of combined Rosemary and Oil and season with salt and pepper.
Put the prepared lamb into the basket of your Air Fryer and set to 2000C for the first 15 minutes.

Reset to 1600C for a further one hour and 15 minutes for a well done roast. Serve immediately and Enjoy!

Za'atar Lamb Chops

Preparation Time: 5 minutes
Cooking time: 10 minutes
Overall time: 15 minutes
Servings: 2 to 4 people
Recipe **Ingredients:**
8 lamb loin chops, trimmed
3 cloves of garlic, crushed
1 tsp. of extra-virgin olive oil
½ fresh lemon
1 ¼ tsp. of kosher salt
1 tablespoon of Za'atar
Fresh ground pepper, to taste
Direction:
Rub the lamb chops with oil and garlic. Squeeze the lemon over both sides, then season with salt, zatar and black pepper.
Preheat the air fryer to 4000F. In batches in an even layer, cook to desired liking, about 4 to 5 minutes on each side.
My chops had 2 ½ ounces of raw meat on each bone, nutritional info is based off of that.

Braised Lamb Shanks

Preparation Time: 5 minutes
Cooking time: 20 minutes
Servings: 2 to 4 people
Recipe **Ingredients:**
4 lamb shanks
1½ tsp. of kosher salt
½ tsp. of freshly ground black pepper
4 garlic cloves, crushed
2 tbsp. of olive oil 4 to 6 sprigs fresh rosemary
3 cups of beef broth, divided
2 tbsp. of balsamic vinegar
Direction:
Rub the lamb shanks with the salt and pepper and place on the Baking pan. Take the smashed garlic and rub well over the lamb.
Coat the seasoned shanks with the olive oil and place the rosemary around and underneath the lamb.
Put the prepared pan with the lamb into rack Position Select Dual Cook. First, set to Roast at 425°F for 20 minutes, and then to Low at 250°F for 2 hours.
Turn the lamb once while roasting. Add 2 cups of the broth and vinegar when oven switches to Low.
Add remaining broth with 1 hour of cooking time remaining. Lamb is done when it easily pulls away from the bone. Serve immediately and Enjoy!

Pork Cutlets

Preparation Time: 10 minutes
Cooking time: 10 minutes
Servings: 2 to 4 people
Recipe **Ingredients:**
1 pound of boneless pork chops
¼ cup of all-purpose flour
½ teaspoon of salt
¼ teaspoon of pepper
2 eggs
¾ cup of panko breadcrumbs
honey Dijon dipping sauce
2 tablespoon mayonnaise
2 teaspoon of Dijon
½ teaspoon of apple cider vinegar
2 teaspoon of honey
Dash of salt
Direction:
Between two layers on saran wrap, evenly pound the pork chops until they are ¼ inch thick.
Add the flour, salt and pepper to a large plate and stir with a fork until well combined.
In a medium bowl, whisk the two eggs. On a separate plate add the Panko breadcrumbs. Dip each pork cutlet into the flour, shaking off any excess.
Then dip the floured pork into the egg wash. Finally, dip the pork into the breadcrumbs. Press the meat into the breadcrumbs so there is a good coating.
Arrange the cutlets in the Air fryer and cook at 3900F for about 10 to 12 minutes, or until the pork reaches an internal temperature of 1650F.
Meanwhile, prepare the honey Dijon dipping sauce, but stirring all of the **Ingredients:** together. Serve the cooked pork with the sauce.

Panko Crusted Pork Chops

Preparation Time: 10 minutes
Cooking time: 12 minutes
Overall time: 22 minutes
Servings: 2 to 4 people
Recipe **Ingredients:**
¼ tsp. of salt
2 to 4 center cut boneless pork chops excess fat trimmed
1 egg beaten
1 cup of panko
1 tbsp. of Parmesan cheese
1 ½ tsp. of paprika
½ tsp. of granulated garlic
½ tsp. of onion powder
½ tsp. of chili powder
¼ tsp. of pepper
Direction:
Preheat air fryer to 400 degrees while you prepare the pork chops.
Sprinkle pork chops with salt on both sides and let sit while you prepare the seasonings and egg wash. Place beaten egg in a shallow medium bowl.

In another shallow medium bowl, combine panko, Parmesan cheese, paprika, garlic, onion powder, chili powder, and pepper.
Dip the pork chops in the egg, followed by the panko mixture. Place in the hot air fryer basket and spray with oil. Cook at 4000F for about 12 minutes.
Flip the pork chops over after 6 minutes, spray with more oil and continue cooking for the remaining 6 minutes.
Serves immediately and Enjoy!

BBQ Pork Ribs

Preparation Time: 5 minutes
Cooking time: 35 minutes

Servings: 2 to 4 people
Recipe **Ingredients:**
1 tbsp. of kosher salt
1 tbsp. of dark brown sugar
1 tbsp. of sweet paprika
1 tsp. of garlic powder
1 tsp. of onion powder
1 tsp. of poultry seasoning
½ tsp. of mustard powder
1/2 tsp. of freshly ground black pepper
2 ¼ lb. of individually cut st. louis–style pork spareribs
Direction:
In a large bowl, whisk together the salt, brown sugar, paprika, garlic powder, onion powder, poultry seasoning, mustard powder, and pepper.
Add the ribs and toss and rub the seasonings into them with your hands until they're fully coated.
Arrange the ribs in the air fryer basket standing up on their ends and leaned up against the wall of the basket and each other.
Cook at 350°F until the ribs are tender inside and golden brown and crisp on the outside, for about 35 minutes.
Transfer the ribs to plates and serve hot.

Spicy Pork Chop

Preparation Time: 20 Minutes
Servings: 4
Ingredients:
Onion powder – 2 tbsp.
Dried Oregano – 2 tbsp.
Dried rosemary – 1 tbsp.
Olive Oil – 1 tbsp.
Ground cumin - 1 tbsp.
Garlic powder – 2 tbsp.
Sweet Paprika – 2 tbsp.
Salt and black pepper
Pork chops – 4 medium
Directions:
Get a bowl, mix in the dried rosemary, oregano, Sweet Paprika, olive oil, garlic, cumin, salt and pepper and rub the pork chops well
Put the pork chops in your air fryer's basket and cook for 15 minutes at 400°F, and ensure you flip halfway

Share between plates
Serve and enjoy while warm
Nutrition:
Calories 281, Fiber 7, Protein 19, carbs 17, Fat 18

Chinese Pork and Broccoli Stir Fry Recipe

Preparation Time: 20 Minutes
Servings: 4
Ingredients:
Oyster sauce – ½ cup
Olive oil – 2 tsp
Broccoli florets – 1 pound
Soy sauce – 1 tsp
Minced garlic clove – 1
Pork stew meat – 1 pound
Directions:
Get a bowl, mix in the oyster sauce, olive oil, broccoli forest, soy sauce, pork stew meat, garlic clove and stir well
Place the mixture in an air fryer and cook for 15 minutes at 390°F
Divide into bowls and share
Serve and enjoy
Nutrition:
Fat 12, Protein 20, Calories 281, Carbs 19, Fiber 7

French-Style Onion Beef

Preparation Time: 20 Minutes
Servings: 2
Ingredients:
Olive oil – 1 tbsp.
Green bell pepper cut into strips – 1
Mustard – ½ tbsp.
Provencal herbs – 2 tsps.
Sliced red onion – 1
Salt and black pepper
Beef fillets cut into strips – 7 ounces
Directions:
Put all your **Ingredients:** olive oil, green bell pepper, mustard, sliced red onion, Provencal herbs, beef fillets, salt and black pepper in a baking dish that suits your air fryer and mix well
Put the pan on the fryer and cook for 15 minutes at 400°F
Share the mixture between bowls and enjoy
Nutrition:
Protein 20, Calories 291, Fat 8, Fiber 7, Carbs 19

Simple Beef and Mushroom Mix

Preparation Time: 20 Minutes
Servings: 2
Ingredients:
Chopped yellow onion – 1
Cut into streaks, beef steaks – 2
Sliced white mushrooms – 8 ounces
Salt and black pepper

Dark soy sauce – 2 tbsp
Olive oil – 1 tsp

Directions:

Get a baking dish that suits your air fryer, mix in the onion, beef steaks, mushrooms, soy sauce, olive oil, salt and pepper and stir well
Arrange the pan in the air fryer and cook for 17 minutes at 390°F
Share everything between plates
Enjoy while hot

Nutrition:

Fat 8, Protein 20, Calories 285, Carbs 18, Fiber 2

Tasty Oregano Pork Chops

Preparation Time: 20 Minutes
Servings: 4

Ingredients:

Pork chops – 4
Minced garlic cloves 4
Salt and Pepper
Chopped Oregano – 2 tablespoon
Olive oil – 2 tbsp

Directions:

Get a bowl and combine the pork chops, garlic, salt, pepper, oregano, olive oil and mix thoroughly
Arrange the chops to your air fryer's basket and cook for 15 minutes at 400°F
Serve with a side salad and enjoy

Nutrition:

Fat 7, Protein 22, Calories 301, Fiber 5, Carbs 19

Garlic Crusted Rack of lamb

Preparation Time: 30 Minutes
Servings: 4

Ingredients:

Vegetable oil – 1 tbsp
Whisked egg – 1
Salt and black pepper
Minced garlic cloves – 2
Toasted and crushed Macedonia nuts – 2 tbsp
Chopped Oregano – 1 tbsp
Rack of lamb – 28 ounces

Directions:

Get a bowl, mix in the pepper, salt, Oil and garlic; ensure you rub the lamb well
In a separate bowl, mix in the Macedonia nut with the salt, pepper and Oregano
Place the egg in a third bowl
Firstly, dredge the lamb in the egg and then in the Macedonia nuts mix
Arrange the lamb in an air fryer basket and cook for 10 minutes at 380°F
Share between plates and serve

Nutrition:

Carbs 20, Calories 280, Protein 19, Fiber 8, Fat 12

Coconut-Pork Stir Fry

Preparation Time: 20 Minutes
Servings: 4
Ingredients:
Minced garlic cloves – 2
Chilli paste – 2 tsps.
Soy sauce – 3 tbsps.
Coconut milk - 7 ounces
Salt and black pepper
Chilli paste – 2 tsps.
Chopped shallot – 1
Cut into strips, pork chops – 14 ounces
Olive Oil – 2 tbsps.
Grated ginger – 1 tsp
Directions:
Get a baking dish that suits your fryer, add in the pork, chilli paste, ginger, shallots, pepper, Oil, soy sauce, salt and pepper and stir well
Put the pan in an air fryer and cook for 12 minutes at 400°F, shaking the fryer halfway
Put in the coconut milk, stir and cook for an additional 4 minutes
Share everything in the bowls and serve
Nutrition:
Fat 11, Protein 14, Calories 283, Carbs 22, Fiber 9

Creamy Sprouts and Pork

Preparation Time: 30 Minutes
Servings: 4
Ingredients:
Sour cream – ½ cup
Cubed tenderloin – 1 pound pork
Trimmed Brussels Sprouts – 1½ pound
Olive Oil – 2 tbsps.
Chopped rosemary – 2 tbsps.
Minced garlic clove – 1
Salt and pepper
Directions:
Get a pan that suits your air fryer, mix in the pork with the rosemary, garlic, salt, pepper, Oil and stir well
Put the pan in an air fryer and cook for 17 minutes at 400°F
Add the sprout and the sour cream and stir thoroughly
Put the pan on the air fryer and cook for an additional 8 minutes
Share everything into bowls and serve
Nutrition:
Fat 13, Calories 280, Protein 18, Fiber 9, Carbs 22

Pork and Chives Dumpling

Preparation Time: 32 Minutes
Servings: 6
Ingredients:
Chopped chives – 2 tbsps.
Salt and black pepper

Mustard – 2 tbsps.
Chopped tarragon – ¼ cup
Cubed tenderloin pork – 1 pound
Mayonnaise – 1 cup
Minced cloves – 2 garlic
Directions:
Put mustard, tarragon, chives, pork, garlic, salt and pepper into the pan that suits your air fryer, stir well
Arrange the pan in the air fryer and cook for 15 minutes at 400°F
Put the mayo and stir
Put the pan in the air fryer for an additional 7 minutes
Share in a bowl and serve
Nutrition:
Fiber 2, Calories 280, Protein 14, Carbs 17, fat 12

Beef with Red wine sauce

Preparation Time: 50 Minutes
Servings: 6
Ingredients:
Minced garlic cloves – 3
Beef roast – 3 pounds
Red wine – ¾ cup
Salt and pepper
Melted butter – 2 tbsps.
Beef stock – 1¾ cups
Mustard – 1 tbsp.
Directions:
Get a bowl, mix in the beef with butter, garlic, pepper, salt and mustard, rub the meet thoroughly
Place the beef roast in your air fryer and cook for 15 minutes at 400°F
Get a pan over medium-high heat and add the stock and the wine
After then add the beef roast and put the pan in the air fryer, cook for 25 minutes at 380°F
Share into bowls and serve
Nutrition:
Calories 300, Carbs 18, Protein 22, Fiber 4, Fat 11

Paprika Lamb chops and dill

Preparation Time: 30 Minutes
Servings: 6
Ingredients:
Minced garlic clove – 1
Salt and pepper
Chopped dill – 2 tbsps.
Olive Oil – 1 tbsps.
Chopped yellow onions – 2
Chicken stocks-3 cups
Sweet Paprika – 2 tbsps.
Chops lamb – 1 pound
Heavy cream – 1½ cups
Directions:
Arrange the lamb chops in your air fryer, add pepper, salt, Paprika, garlic and rub the chops thoroughly

Cook for 10 minutes at 380°F
Take the lamb to a baking dish that suits your air fryer
Add the onions, cream, dill, stock and stir
Put the pan in the fryer and cook for an additional 8 minutes
Share within plates and serve hot
Nutrition:
Fiber 10, Protein 25, Carbs 19, Calories 310, Fat 8

Pork Chops with Mustard Sauce

Preparation Time: 25 Minutes
Servings: 6
Ingredients:
Olive Oil – ¼ cup
Salt and pepper
Mustard – 1 tbsps.
Olive Oil – ¼ cup
Minced garlic cloves – 2
Sweet Paprika – 1 tsp
Directions:
Mix all **Ingredients:** in a bowl and coat the pork chops well
Arrange the pork chops to your air fryer's basket and cook for 15 minutes at 400°F
Share the chops between plates and serve
Nutrition:
Carbs 17, Protein 28, Calories 284, Fat 14, Fiber 4

Beef Roast and Red Grapes

Preparation Time: 50 Minutes
Servings: 4
Ingredients:
Chopped red onion – 1
Red grapes – ½ pound
Chopped thyme – 1 tsp
Olive Oil – 3 tbsps.
Salt and pepper
Chicken stock – 1½ cups
Red grapes – ½ pound
Cubed, beef roast meat – 1 pound
Dry white wine – ½ cup
Directions:
Get a pan that suits your air fryer, place over a medium-high heat
Put the salt, beef and pepper, stir and brown for 5 minutes
Put the stock, garlic, thyme, onions, toss and cook for 7 minutes
Arrange the pan to your air fryer and cook for 25 minutes at 390°F
Add the grapes, stir gently and cook everything for 6 more minutes
Share between plates and serve right away
Nutrition:
Fat 12, Protein 28, Calories 290, Fiber 5, Carbs 19

Sage Pork Chop Recipe

Preparation Time: 60 Minutes
Servings: 6
Ingredients:
Dried Oregano – 1 tsp
Dried sage – 3 tsp
Garlic powder – ½ tsp
Beef stock – ¾ cup
Boneless and cubed pork loin – 2 ½ pounds
Olive Oil – 2 tbsps.
Smoked Paprika – ½ tsp
Salt and pepper
Directions:
Get an oil that suits your air fryer, put Oil and place over a medium heat
Add the pork, stir and brown for 5 minutes
Add the garlic, Oregano, pepper, Paprika, sage, basil and pepper, toss and stir for 2 minutes
Add the stock and toss
Put the pan on the fryer and cook for 40 minutes at 360°F
Divide everything between plates and serve
Nutrition:
Protein 29, Calories 290, Fiber 6, Fat 11, Carbs 20

Beef Roast Recipe

Preparation Time: 65 Minutes
Servings: 6
Ingredients:
Salt and pepper
Olive Oil – 3 tbsps.
Minced garlic – 3 tbsps.
Beef roast – 2 pounds
Smoked Paprika – 1 tbsp
Olive Oil – 3 tbsps.
Directions:
Get a bowl,
Mix in the beef roast, garlic, paprika, oil, salt and pepper and toss to coat well
Put the roast in your air fryer and cook for 55 minutes at 390°F
Slice the roast, divide it between plates and serve with a side salad
Nutrition:
Fiber 9, Calories 291, Protein 26, Carbs 20, Fat 12

Pork Loin Terragon

Preparation Time: 65 Minutes
Servings: 6
Ingredients:
sweet Paprika – 2 tsps.
Trimmed pork loin – 3 pounds
minced garlic cloves
Chopped tarragon – 2 tablespoons
Salt and pepper
Olive Oil – ¼ cup

Directions:
Get a bowl and mix all the **Ingredients:**, rub well
Arrange the roast to your air fryer and cook for 15 minutes at 390°F
Slice the roasts.
Divide between plates and serve
Nutrition:
Fat 14, Calories 290, Protein 22, Fiber 9, Carbs 19

Beef and Celery Stir-Fry

Preparation Time: 65 Minutes
Servings: 6
Ingredients:
Beef roast – 3 cups
Canned tomatoes – 16 ounces
Chopped celery – 1 pound
Olive oil – 2 tbsps.
Chopped yellow onion
Salt and black pepper
Beef stock – 3 cups
Directions:
Put all the beef roast, beef stock, celery, olive oil, onion, tomatoes, salt and pepper baking dish that suits your air fryer and mix well
Place the pan in the fryer and cook for 55 minutes at 390°F
Slice the roast, divide it and the celery and ensure you mix between plates
Serve and enjoy
Nutrition:
Fat 12, Protein 20, Calories 300, Fiber 4, Carbs 18

Asian Beef Mix

Preparation Time: 25 Minutes
Servings: 4
Ingredients:
Chopped green onion – 1 cup
Toasted sesame seed – ¼ cup
Soy sauce – 1 cup
Minced garlic cloves – 5
Beef stew meat – 1 pound
Black pepper
Directions:
Get a pan that fits your air fryer.
Add the onion, sesame seed, soy sauce, garlic cloves, stew meat, black pepper and mix well
Place the pan in the air fryer and cook for 20 minutes at 390°F
Share everything into bowls and serve
Nutrition:
Carbs 20, Protein 19, Calories 289, Fiber 12, Fat 8

Pork and Pepper Stir Fry

Preparation Time: 25 Minutes
Servings: 4
Ingredients:
Olive Oil – 2 tbsps.

Chopped shallot – 4
Fish sauce – 2 tbsps.
Salt and black pepper – A pinch
Cut in strips; red bell pepper – 2
Minced garlic cloves – 4
Cut into strips; pound pork – 1
Beef stock - 1/2 cup

Directions:

Get a pan that suits your fryer
Put the olive oil, shallot, fish, bell pepper, garlic, pound pork, beef stock and stir
Put the pan in an air fryer and cook for 20 minutes at 400°F
Share everything within plates and serve

Nutrition:

Calories 293, Protein 29, Fiber 12, Carbs 20,Fat 12

Slow-Cooked Lamb with Beans

Preparation Time: 35 Minutes
Servings: 4
Ingredients:

Cubed lamb coin – 8 ounces
Grated ginger – 1 tbsps.
Sliced yellow onion – 1
Olive oil – ½ tsp
Salt and black pepper
drained, canned kidney beans – 3 ounces
Soy sauce – 3 tbsps.
Minced garlic clove – 1
Chopped carrot – 1
Soy sauce – 3 tbsps.
Cubed lamb coin – 8 ounces

Directions:

Get a baking dish that suits your air fryer, add up all the **Ingredients:** and mix well
Put the dish in the air fryer and cook for 30 minutes at 390°F
Share everything into bowls and serve

Nutrition:

Fat 3, Protein 18, Calories 275, Carbs 20, Fiber 7

Pork chops with Lemon Spinach

Preparation Time: 20 Minutes
Servings: 4
Ingredients:

Salt and black pepper
Pork chops – 2
Spinach pesto – 3 tbsps.
Beef stock – ½ cup
Baby spinach – 2 cups

Directions:

Put the pork chops, pepper, salt and spinach in a bowl and stir thoroughly
Put the pork chops in the air fryer and cook for 4 minutes on each side at 400°F
Arrange the chops to a pan that suits your air fryer
Add the stock and baby spinach

Place the pan in the fryer and cook for 7 minutes at 400°F
Share everything between plates and serve
Nutrition:
Protein 1Calories Carbs 2Fat 11, Fiber 9

Classic Ground Beef Mix

Preparation Time: 25 Minutes
Servings: 4
Ingredients:
Ground beef – 1 pound
Salt and pepper
Olive oil – 1 tbsps.
Cumin – ½ tsp
Minced garlic cloves – 2
Chopped green bell pepper
Chopped yellow onion
Tomato Salsa – ¼ cup
Directions:
Heat the pan that suits your air fryer over a medium heat
Put the onion, bell peppers, garlic and cumin and cook for 3 minutes
Put the meat, stir and cook for 3 minutes and take off the heat
Add the Salsa, stir and place the pan in the fryer
Cook for 14 minutes at 380°F
Serve and enjoy
Nutrition:
Protein 16, Calories 264, Carbs 20, Fat 11, Fiber 4

Delicious Smoked Pork Roast

Preparation Time: 60 Minutes
Servings: 4
Ingredients:
Chopped Oregano – 2 tbsps.
Smoked Paprika – 3 tbsps.
Salt and black pepper
Pork loin roast – 2 pounds
Brown sugar – 1 tbsps.
Olive oil – 1 tbsps.
Liquid smoke – 1 tsp
Directions:
Place all the **Ingredients:** in a bowl
Mix well and ensure the pork is thoroughly coated
Arrange the roast to your air fryer and cook for 55 minutes at 370°F
Slice the roast, share it between roast and serve
Nutrition:
Fiber 9, Protein 18, Calories 300, Carbs 22, Fat 12

Pork Fillet and Cauli Flower

Preparation Time: 27 Minutes
Servings: 4
Ingredients:
Minced garlic clove – 1

Olive Oil – 2 tbsps.
Cauliflower head, florets separated – 1
Cubed pork stew meat – 1 pound
Sugar – 1 tsp
Balsamic Vinegar – ½ cup
Soy sauce – 1 tsp

Directions:

Put all the **Ingredients:** in a pan that suits your air fryer and mix thoroughly
Put the pan into the fryer and cook for 22 minutes at 390°F
Share into bowls
Serve and enjoy warm

Nutrition:

Protein 20, Calories 270, Fiber 7, Fat 9, Carbs 23

Pork and Peppers

Preparation Time: 32 Minutes
Servings: 2
Ingredients:

Cut in strips, yellow bell pepper – 1
Cut in strips, red bell pepper – 1
Olive Oil – 2 tbsps.
Cut in strips, pork tenderloin – 7 ounces
Chopped sweet onion -1
Salt and black pepper
Cut in pieces, green bell pepper – 1

Directions:

Put all the **Ingredients:** into a pan that suits your air fryer and toss well
Place the pan in an air fryer and cook for 22 minutes at 390°F
Share the mix between plates and serve

Nutrition:

Protein 19, Fiber 7, Calories 280, Fat 13, Carbs 21

Ground Beef and Peas

Preparation Time: 30 Minutes
Servings: 2
Ingredients:

Cut into strips, beef steak – 2
Snow peas – 14 ounces
Olive Oil – 1 tbsps.
Salt and black pepper
Soy sauce – 2 tbsps.

Directions:

Get a pan that suits your air fryer
Add in the olive oil, soy sauce, beef steak, snow peas, salt and pepper
Put the pan in a fryer and cook for 25 minutes at 390°F
Share between plates and serve

Nutrition:

Carbs 22, Fat 11, Calories 265, Protein 19, Fiber 4

Fennel-Crusted Pork Chops

Preparation Time: 20 Minutes
Servings: 4
Ingredients:
Pork chops – 2
Olive oil – 3 tbsps.
Chopped rosemary – 1 tbsps.
Salt and pepper
Roasted seed - tablespoon fennel
Directions:
Get a bowl, add in the pork chops with the salt, fennel, Oil, pepper and the rosemary
Stir and ensure the pork chops are coated well
Arrange the chops to your air fryer and cook for 15 minutes at 400°F
Share the chops between plates and serve
Nutrition:
Fat 11, Protein 20, Calories 281, Fiber 8, Carbs 17

Lamb Meatballs with Lemon Zest

Preparation Time: 22 Minutes
Servings: 8
Ingredients:
Salt and black pepper
Whisked egg – 1
Cooking spray
Lemon zest – ½ tbsps.
Oregano chopped – 1 tbsps.
Minced lamb meat – 4 ounces
Directions:
Get a bowl, combine all the **Ingredients:** except the cooking spray and stir well
Shape the medium-sized meatballs out of the mix
Arrange the meatballs in your air fryer's basket
Grease them with cooking spray and cook for 12 minutes at 400°F
Share between plates and serve
Nutrition:
Carbs 22, Protein 19, Calories 294, Fat 12, Fiber 2

Favorite Pork Meatloaf

Preparation Time: 25 Minutes
Servings: 4
Ingredients:
Cooking spray
Chopped thyme - 1 tbsps.
Chopped chorizo – 1 ounce
Salt and black pepper
Ground pork meat – 1 pound
Chopped yellow onion – 1
Whisked egg – 1
Breadcrumbs – 3 tbsps.
Directions:
Get a bowl and mix all the **Ingredients:** except the cooking spray

Stir and combine well
Transfer the mixture to a loaf pan that fits your air fryer and grease with Oil
Arrange the pan in the air fryer and cook for 20 minutes at 390°F
Slice and serve
Nutrition:
Carbs 19, Protein 26, Calories 290, Fat 12, Fiber 1

Easy Pork Steaks

Preparation Time: 19 Minutes
Servings: 4
Ingredients:
Pork steaks – 4
Melted butter – 1 tbsps.
Salt and black pepper
Sweet Paprika – 1 tbsps.
Directions:
Rub the pork steaks with butter, salt, pepper, Paprika until it's thoroughly coated
Arrange the steaks to your air fryer's basket and cook for 7 minutes at 390°F on each side
Share the steaks between plates and serve
Nutrition:
Calories 250, Protein 21, Carbs 18, Fat 12, Fiber 5

Homemade Sausage Mix

Preparation Time: 25 Minutes
Servings: 4
Ingredients:
Sliced red onion – 1
Sliced red onion – 1
Chopped rosemary – 1 tbsps.
Halved sausage link – 6 pork
Sweet Paprika – 1 tbsps.
Salt and black pepper
Minced garlic cloves – 2
Directions:
Get a pan that suits your air fryer, mix all the air fryer and stir
Put the pan in the fryer and cook for 20 minutes at 360°F
Share between plates and serve
Nutrition:
Protein 18, Fiber 7, Calories 280, Fat 11, Carbs 18

Spicy Pork Chop

Preparation Time: 20 Minutes
Servings: 4
Ingredients:
Onion powder – 2 tbsp.
Dried Oregano – 2 tbsp.
Dried rosemary – 1 tbsp.
Olive Oil – 1 tbsp.
Ground cumin - 1 tbsp.
Garlic powder – 2 tbsp.
Sweet Paprika – 2 tbsp.

Salt and black pepper
Pork chops – 4 medium
Directions:
Get a bowl, mix in the dried rosemary, oregano, Sweet Paprika, olive oil, garlic, cumin, salt and pepper and rub the pork chops well
Put the pork chops in your air fryer's basket and cook for 15 minutes at 400°F, and ensure you flip halfway
Share between plates
Serve and enjoy while warm
Nutrition:
Calories 281, Fiber 7, Protein 19, carbs 17, Fat 18

Chinese Pork and Broccoli Stir Fry Recipe

Preparation Time: 20 Minutes
Servings: 4
Ingredients:
Oyster sauce – ½ cup
Olive oil – 2 tsp
Broccoli florets – 1 pound
Soy sauce – 1 tsp
Minced garlic clove – 1
Pork stew meat – 1 pound
Directions:
Get a bowl, mix in the oyster sauce, olive oil, broccoli forest, soy sauce, pork stew meat, garlic clove and stir well
Place the mixture in an air fryer and cook for 15 minutes at 390°F
Divide into bowls and share
Serve and enjoy
Nutrition:
Fat 12, Protein 20, Calories 281, Carbs 19, Fiber 7

French-Style Onion Beef

Preparation Time: 20 Minutes
Servings: 2
Ingredients:
Olive oil – 1 tbsp.
Green bell pepper cut into strips – 1
Mustard – ½ tbsp.
Provencal herbs – 2 tsps.
Sliced red onion – 1
Salt and black pepper
Beef fillets cut into strips – 7 ounces
Directions:
Put all your **Ingredients:** olive oil, green bell pepper, mustard, sliced red onion, Provencal herbs, beef fillets, salt and black pepper in a baking dish that suits your air fryer and mix well
Put the pan on the fryer and cook for 15 minutes at 400°F
Share the mixture between bowls and enjoy
Nutrition:
Protein 20, Calories 291, Fat 8, Fiber 7, Carbs 19

Simple Beef and Mushroom Mix

Preparation Time: 20 Minutes
Servings: 2
Ingredients:
Chopped yellow onion – 1
Cut into streaks, beef steaks – 2
Sliced white mushrooms – 8 ounces
Salt and black pepper
Dark soy sauce – 2 tbsp
Olive oil – 1 tsp
Directions:
Get a baking dish that suits your air fryer, mix in the onion, beef steaks, mushrooms, soy sauce, olive oil, salt and pepper and stir well
Arrange the pan in the air fryer and cook for 17 minutes at 390°F
Share everything between plates
Enjoy while hot
Nutrition:
Fat 8, Protein 20, Calories 285, Carbs 18, Fiber 2

Tasty Oregano Pork Chops

Preparation Time: 20 Minutes
Servings: 4
Ingredients:
Pork chops – 4
Minced garlic cloves 4
Salt and Pepper
Chopped Oregano – 2 tablespoon
Olive oil – 2 tbsp
Directions:
Get a bowl and combine the pork chops, garlic, salt, pepper, oregano, olive oil and mix thoroughly
Arrange the chops to your air fryer's basket and cook for 15 minutes at 400°F
Serve with a side salad and enjoy
Nutrition:
Fat 7, Protein 22, Calories 301, Fiber 5, Carbs 19

Garlic Crusted Rack of lamb

Preparation Time: 30 Minutes
Servings: 4
Ingredients:
Vegetable oil – 1 tbsp
Whisked egg – 1
Salt and black pepper
Minced garlic cloves – 2
Toasted and crushed Macedonia nuts – 2 tbsp
Chopped Oregano – 1 tbsp
Rack of lamb – 28 ounces
Directions:
Get a bowl, mix in the pepper, salt, Oil and garlic; ensure you rub the lamb well
In a separate bowl, mix in the Macedonia nut with the salt, pepper and Oregano

Place the egg in a third bowl
Firstly, dredge the lamb in the egg and then in the Macedonia nuts mix
Arrange the lamb in an air fryer basket and cook for 10 minutes at 380°F
Share between plates and serve

Nutrition:

Carbs 20, Calories 280, Protein 19, Fiber 8, Fat 12

Coconut-Pork Stir Fry

Preparation Time: 20 Minutes

Servings: 4

Ingredients:

Minced garlic cloves – 2
Chilli paste – 2 tsps.
Soy sauce – 3 tbsps.
Coconut milk - 7 ounces
Salt and black pepper
Chilli paste – 2 tsps.
Chopped shallot – 1
Cut into strips, pork chops – 14 ounces
Olive Oil – 2 tbsps.
Grated ginger – 1 tsp

Directions:

Get a baking dish that suits your fryer, add in the pork, chilli paste, ginger, shallots, pepper, Oil, soy sauce, salt and pepper and stir well
Put the pan in an air fryer and cook for 12 minutes at 400°F, shaking the fryer halfway
Put in the coconut milk, stir and cook for an additional 4 minutes
Share everything in the bowls and serve

Nutrition:

Fat 11, Protein 14, Calories 283, Carbs 22, Fiber 9

Creamy Sprouts and Pork

Preparation Time: 30 Minutes

Servings: 4

Ingredients:

Sour cream – ½ cup
Cubed tenderloin – 1 pound pork
Trimmed Brussels Sprouts – 1½ pound
Olive Oil – 2 tbsps.
Chopped rosemary – 2 tbsps.
Minced garlic clove – 1
Salt and pepper

Directions:

Get a pan that suits your air fryer, mix in the pork with the rosemary, garlic, salt, pepper, Oil and stir well
Put the pan in an air fryer and cook for 17 minutes at 400°F
Add the sprout and the sour cream and stir thoroughly
Put the pan on the air fryer and cook for an additional 8 minutes
Share everything into bowls and serve

Nutrition:

Fat 13, Calories 280, Protein 18, Fiber 9, Carbs 22

Pork and Chives Dumpling

Preparation Time: 32 Minutes
Servings: 6
Ingredients:
Chopped chives – 2 tbsps.
Salt and black pepper
Mustard – 2 tbsps.
Chopped tarragon – ¼ cup
Cubed tenderloin pork – 1 pound
Mayonnaise – 1 cup
Minced cloves – 2 garlic
Directions:
Put mustard, tarragon, chives, pork, garlic, salt and pepper into the pan that suits your air fryer, stir well
Arrange the pan in the air fryer and cook for 15 minutes at 400°F
Put the mayo and stir
Put the pan in the air fryer for an additional 7 minutes
Share in a bowl and serve
Nutrition:
Fiber 2, Calories 280, Protein 14, Carbs 17, fat 12

Beef with Red wine sauce

Preparation Time: 50 Minutes
Servings: 6
Ingredients:
Minced garlic cloves – 3
Beef roast – 3 pounds
Red wine – ¾ cup
Salt and pepper
Melted butter – 2 tbsps.
Beef stock – 1¾ cups
Mustard – 1 tbsp.
Directions:
Get a bowl, mix in the beef with butter, garlic, pepper, salt and mustard, rub the meet thoroughly
Place the beef roast in your air fryer and cook for 15 minutes at 400°F
Get a pan over medium-high heat and add the stock and the wine
After then add the beef roast and put the pan in the air fryer, cook for 25 minutes at 380°F
Share into bowls and serve
Nutrition:
Calories 300, Carbs 18, Protein 22, Fiber 4, Fat 11

Paprika Lamb chops and dill

Preparation Time: 30 Minutes
Servings: 6
Ingredients:
Minced garlic clove – 1
Salt and pepper
Chopped dill – 2 tbsps.
Olive Oil – 1 tbsps.
Chopped yellow onions – 2

Chicken stocks-3 cups
Sweet Paprika – 2 tbsps.
Chops lamb – 1 pound
Heavy cream – 1½ cups
Directions:
Arrange the lamb chops in your air fryer, add pepper, salt, Paprika, garlic and rub the chops thoroughly
Cook for 10 minutes at 380°F
Take the lamb to a baking dish that suits your air fryer
Add the onions, cream, dill, stock and stir
Put the pan in the fryer and cook for an additional 8 minutes
Share within plates and serve hot
Nutrition:
Fiber 10, Protein 25, Carbs 19, Calories 310, Fat 8

Pork Chops with Mustard Sauce

Preparation Time: 25 Minutes
Servings: 6
Ingredients:
Olive Oil – ¼ cup
Salt and pepper
Mustard – 1 tbsps.
Olive Oil – ¼ cup
Minced garlic cloves – 2
Sweet Paprika – 1 tsp
Directions:
Mix all **Ingredients:** in a bowl and coat the pork chops well
Arrange the pork chops to your air fryer's basket and cook for 15 minutes at 400°F
Share the chops between plates and serve
Nutrition:
Carbs 17, Protein 28, Calories 284, Fat 14, Fiber 4

Beef Roast and Red Grapes

Preparation Time: 50 Minutes
Servings: 4
Ingredients:
Chopped red onion – 1
Red grapes – ½ pound
Chopped thyme – 1 tsp
Olive Oil – 3 tbsps.
Salt and pepper
Chicken stock – 1½ cups
Red grapes – ½ pound
Cubed, beef roast meat – 1 pound
Dry white wine – ½ cup
Directions:
Get a pan that suits your air fryer, place over a medium-high heat
Put the salt, beef and pepper, stir and brown for 5 minutes
Put the stock, garlic, thyme, onions, toss and cook for 7 minutes
Arrange the pan to your air fryer and cook for 25 minutes at 390°F
Add the grapes, stir gently and cook everything for 6 more minutes

Share between plates and serve right away

Nutrition:

Fat 12, Protein 28, Calories 290, Fiber 5, Carbs 19

Sage Pork Chop Recipe

Preparation Time: 60 Minutes

Servings: 6

Ingredients:

Dried Oregano – 1 tsp

Dried sage – 3 tsp

Garlic powder – ½ tsp

Beef stock – ¾ cup

Boneless and cubed pork loin – 2 ½ pounds

Olive Oil – 2 tbsps.

Smoked Paprika – ½ tsp

Salt and pepper

Directions:

Get an oil that suits your air fryer, put Oil and place over a medium heat

Add the pork, stir and brown for 5 minutes

Add the garlic, Oregano, pepper, Paprika, sage, basil and pepper, toss and stir for 2 minutes

Add the stock and toss

Put the pan on the fryer and cook for 40 minutes at 360°F

Divide everything between plates and serve

Nutrition:

Protein 29, Calories 290, Fiber 6, Fat 11, Carbs 20

Beef Roast Recipe

Preparation Time: 65 Minutes

Servings: 6

Ingredients:

Salt and pepper

Olive Oil – 3 tbsps.

Minced garlic – 3 tbsps.

Beef roast – 2 pounds

Smoked Paprika – 1 tbsp

Olive Oil – 3 tbsps.

Directions:

Get a bowl,

Mix in the beef roast, garlic, paprika, oil, salt and pepper and toss to coat well

Put the roast in your air fryer and cook for 55 minutes at 390°F

Slice the roast, divide it between plates and serve with a side salad

Nutrition:

Fiber 9, Calories 291, Protein 26, Carbs 20, Fat 12

Pork Loin Terragon

Preparation Time: 65 Minutes

Servings: 6

Ingredients:

sweet Paprika – 2 tsps.

Trimmed pork loin – 3 pounds

minced garlic cloves

Chopped tarragon – 2 tablespoons
Salt and pepper
Olive Oil – ¼ cup
Directions:
Get a bowl and mix all the **Ingredients:**, rub well
Arrange the roast to your air fryer and cook for 15 minutes at 390°F
Slice the roasts.
Divide between plates and serve
Nutrition:
Fat 14, Calories 290, Protein 22, Fiber 9, Carbs 19

Beef and Celery Stir-Fry

Preparation Time: 65 Minutes
Servings: 6
Ingredients:
Beef roast – 3 cups
Canned tomatoes – 16 ounces
Chopped celery – 1 pound
Olive oil – 2 tbsps.
Chopped yellow onion
Salt and black pepper
Beef stock – 3 cups
Directions:
Put all the beef roast, beef stock, celery, olive oil, onion, tomatoes, salt and pepper baking dish that suits your air fryer and mix well
Place the pan in the fryer and cook for 55 minutes at 390°F
Slice the roast, divide it and the celery and ensure you mix between plates
Serve and enjoy
Nutrition:
Fat 12, Protein 20, Calories 300, Fiber 4, Carbs 18

Asian Beef Mix

Preparation Time: 25 Minutes
Servings: 4
Ingredients:
Chopped green onion – 1 cup
Toasted sesame seed – ¼ cup
Soy sauce – 1 cup
Minced garlic cloves – 5
Beef stew meat – 1 pound
Black pepper
Directions:
Get a pan that fits your air fryer.
Add the onion, sesame seed, soy sauce, garlic cloves, stew meat, black pepper and mix well
Place the pan in the air fryer and cook for 20 minutes at 390°F
Share everything into bowls and serve
Nutrition:
Carbs 20, Protein 19, Calories 289, Fiber 12, Fat 8

Pork and Pepper Stir Fry

Preparation Time: 25 Minutes
Servings: 4
Ingredients:
Olive Oil – 2 tbsps.
Chopped shallot – 4
Fish sauce – 2 tbsps.
Salt and black pepper – A pinch
Cut in strips; red bell pepper – 2
Minced garlic cloves – 4
Cut into strips; pound pork – 1
Beef stock - 1/2 cup
Directions:
Get a pan that suits your fryer
Put the olive oil, shallot, fish, bell pepper, garlic, pound pork, beef stock and stir
Put the pan in an air fryer and cook for 20 minutes at 400°F
Share everything within plates and serve
Nutrition:
Calories 293, Protein 29, Fiber 12, Carbs 20,Fat 12

Slow-Cooked Lamb with Beans

Preparation Time: 35 Minutes
Servings: 4
Ingredients:
Cubed lamb coin – 8 ounces
Grated ginger – 1 tbsps.
Sliced yellow onion – 1
Olive oil – ½ tsp
Salt and black pepper
drained, canned kidney beans – 3 ounces
Soy sauce – 3 tbsps.
Minced garlic clove – 1
Chopped carrot – 1
Soy sauce – 3 tbsps.
Cubed lamb coin – 8 ounces
Directions:
Get a baking dish that suits your air fryer, add up all the **Ingredients:** and mix well
Put the dish in the air fryer and cook for 30 minutes at 390°F
Share everything into bowls and serve
Nutrition:
Fat 3, Protein 18, Calories 275, Carbs 20, Fiber 7

Pork chops with Lemon Spinach

Preparation Time: 20 Minutes
Servings: 4
Ingredients:
Salt and black pepper
Pork chops – 2
Spinach pesto – 3 tbsps.
Beef stock – ½ cup

Baby spinach – 2 cups
Directions:
Put the pork chops, pepper, salt and spinach in a bowl and stir thoroughly
Put the pork chops in the air fryer and cook for 4 minutes on each side at 400°F
Arrange the chops to a pan that suits your air fryer
Add the stock and baby spinach
Place the pan in the fryer and cook for 7 minutes at 400°F
Share everything between plates and serve
Nutrition:
Protein 1Calories Carbs 2Fat 11, Fiber 9

Classic Ground Beef Mix

Preparation Time: 25 Minutes
Servings: 4
Ingredients:
Ground beef – 1 pound
Salt and pepper
Olive oil – 1 tbsps.
Cumin – ½ tsp
Minced garlic cloves – 2
Chopped green bell pepper
Chopped yellow onion
Tomato Salsa – ¼ cup
Directions:
Heat the pan that suits your air fryer over a medium heat
Put the onion, bell peppers, garlic and cumin and cook for 3 minutes
Put the meat, stir and cook for 3 minutes and take off the heat
Add the Salsa, stir and place the pan in the fryer
Cook for 14 minutes at 380°F
Serve and enjoy
Nutrition:
Protein 16, Calories 264, Carbs 20, Fat 11, Fiber 4

FISH & SEAFOOD

Packet Lobster Tail

Preparation Time: 27 minutes
Servings: 2
Ingredients:
2 (6-oz.lobster tails, halved
2 tbsp. salted butter; melted.
1 tsp. dried parsley.
½ tsp. Old Bay seasoning
Juice of ½ medium lemon.
Directions:
Place the two halved tails on a sheet of aluminum foil. Drizzle with butter, Old Bay seasoning and lemon juice.
Seal the foil packets, completely covering tails. Place into the air fryer basket
Adjust the temperature to 375 Degrees F and set the timer for 12 minutes. Once done, sprinkle with dried parsley and serve immediately.
Nutrition: Calories: 234; Protein: 23g; Fiber: 1g; Fat: 19g; Carbs: 7g

Shrimp and Green Beans

Preparation Time: 20 minutes
Servings: 4
Ingredients:
½ lb. green beans; trimmed and halved
1 lb. shrimp; peeled and deveined
¼ cup ghee; melted
2 tbsp. cilantro; chopped.
Juice of 1 lime
A pinch of salt and black pepper
Directions:
In a pan that fits your air fryer, mix all the **Ingredients:**, toss,
Introduce in the fryer and cook at 360°F for 15 minutes shaking the fryer halfway. Divide into bowls and serve
Nutrition: Calories: 222; Fat: 8g; Fiber: 3g; Carbs: 5g; Protein: 10g

Crab Dip

Preparation Time: 18 minutes
Servings: 4
Ingredients:
8 oz. full-fat cream cheese; softened.
2 (6-oz.cans lump crabmeat
¼ cup chopped pickled jalapeños.
¼ cup full-fat sour cream.
¼ cup sliced green onion
½ cup shredded Cheddar cheese
¼ cup full-fat mayonnaise
1 tbsp. lemon juice
½ tsp. hot sauce

Directions:

Place all **Ingredients:** into a 4-cup round baking dish and stir until fully combined. Place dish into the air fryer basket

Adjust the temperature to 400 Degrees F and set the timer for 8 minutes. Dip will be bubbling and hot when done. Serve warm.

Nutrition: Calories: 441; Protein: 18g; Fiber: 6g; Fat: 38g; Carbs: 2g

Sesame Shrimp

Preparation Time: 15 minutes

Servings: 4

Ingredients:

1 lb. shrimp; peeled and deveined

1 tbsp. olive oil

1 tbsp. sesame seeds, toasted

½ tsp. Italian seasoning

A pinch of salt and black pepper

Directions:

Take a bowl and mix the shrimp with the rest of the **Ingredients:** and toss well

Put the shrimp in the air fryer's basket, cook at 370°F for 12 minutes, divide into bowls and serve,

Nutrition: Calories: 199; Fat: 11g; Fiber: 2g; Carbs: 4g; Protein: 11g

Salmon and Cauliflower Rice

Preparation Time: 30 minutes

Servings: 4

Ingredients:

4 salmon fillets; boneless

½ cup chicken stock

1 cup cauliflower, riced

1 tbsp. butter; melted

1 tsp. turmeric powder

Salt and black pepper to taste.

Directions:

In a pan that fits your air fryer, mix the cauliflower rice with the other **Ingredients:** except the salmon and toss

Arrange the salmon fillets over the cauliflower rice, put the pan in the fryer and cook at 360°F for 25 minutes, flipping the fish after 15 minutes

Divide everything between plates and serve

Nutrition: Calories: 241; Fat: 12g; Fiber: 2g; Carbs: 6g; Protein: 12g

Tilapia and Salsa

Preparation Time: 20 minutes

Servings: 4

Ingredients:

4 tilapia fillets; boneless

12 oz. canned tomatoes; chopped.

2 tbsp. green onions; chopped.

2 tbsp. sweet red pepper; chopped.

1 tbsp. balsamic vinegar

1 tbsp. olive oil

A pinch of salt and black pepper

Directions:
Arrange the tilapia in a baking sheet that fits the air fryer and season with salt and pepper.
In a bowl, combine all the other **Ingredients:**, toss and spread over the fish
Introduce the pan in the fryer and cook at 350°F for 15 minutes
Divide the mix between plates and serve.
Nutrition: Calories: 221; Fat: 12g; Fiber: 2g; Carbs: 5g; Protein: 14g

Garlic Tilapia

Preparation Time: 25 minutes
Servings: 4
Ingredients:
4 tilapia fillets; boneless
1 bunch kale; chopped.
2 garlic cloves; minced
3 tbsp. olive oil
1 tsp. fennel seeds
½ tsp. red pepper flakes, crushed
Salt and black pepper to taste.
Directions:
In a pan that fits the fryer, combine all the **Ingredients:**, put the pan in the fryer and cook at 360°F for 20 minutes
Divide everything between plates and serve.
Nutrition: Calories: 240; Fat: 12g; Fiber: 2g; Carbs: 4g; Protein: 12g

Trout and Mint

Preparation Time: 21 minutes
Servings: 4
Ingredients:
1 avocado, peeled, pitted and roughly chopped.
4 rainbow trout
1/3 pine nuts
1 cup olive oil+ 3 tbsp.
1 cup parsley; chopped.
3 garlic cloves; minced
½ cup mint; chopped.
Zest of 1 lemon
Juice of 1 lemon
A pinch of salt and black pepper
Directions:
Pat dry the trout, season with salt and pepper and rub with 3 tbsp. oil
Put the fish in your air fryer's basket and cook for 8 minutes on each side. Divide the fish between plates and drizzle half of the lemon juice all over
In a blender, combine the rest of the oil with the remaining lemon juice, parsley, garlic, mint, lemon zest, pine nuts and the avocado and pulse well. Spread this over the trout and serve.
Nutrition: Calories: 240; Fat: 12g; Fiber: 4g; Carbs: 6g; Protein: 9g

Salmon and Coconut Sauce

Preparation Time: 25 minutes
Servings: 4
Ingredients:
4 salmon fillets; boneless

1/3 cup heavy cream
¼ cup lime juice
½ cup coconut; shredded
¼ cup coconut cream
1 tsp. lime zest; grated
A pinch of salt and black pepper

Directions:

Take a bowl and mix all the **Ingredients:** except the salmon and whisk.

Arrange the fish in a pan that fits your air fryer, drizzle the coconut sauce all over, put the pan in the machine and cook at 360°F for 20 minutes

Divide between plates and serve

Nutrition: Calories: 227; Fat: 12g; Fiber: 2g; Carbs: 4g; Protein: 9g

Simple Salmon

Preparation Time: 22 minutes

Servings: 2

Ingredients:

2 (4-oz.salmon fillets, skin removed
1 medium lemon.
2 tbsp. unsalted butter; melted.
½ tsp. dried dill
½ tsp. garlic powder.

Directions:

Place each fillet on a 5" × 5" square of aluminum foil. Drizzle with butter and sprinkle with garlic powder.

Zest half of the lemon and sprinkle zest over salmon. Slice other half of the lemon and lay two slices on each piece of salmon. Sprinkle dill over salmon

Gather and fold foil at the top and sides to fully close packets. Place foil packets into the air fryer basket. Adjust the temperature to 400 Degrees F and set the timer for 12 minutes

Salmon will be easily flaked and have an internal temperature of at least 145 Degrees F when fully cooked.

Nutrition: Calories: 252; Protein: 29g; Fiber: 4g; Fat: 15g; Carbs: 2g

Cajun Salmon

Preparation Time: 12 minutes

Servings: 2

Ingredients:

2 (4-oz.salmon fillets, skin removed
2 tbsp. unsalted butter; melted.
1 tsp. paprika
¼ tsp. ground black pepper
⅛ tsp. ground cayenne pepper
½ tsp. garlic powder.

Directions:

Brush each fillet with butter. Combine remaining **Ingredients:** in a small bowl and then rub onto fish. Place fillets into the air fryer basket

Adjust the temperature to 390 Degrees F and set the timer for 7 minutes. When fully cooked, internal temperature will be 145 Degrees F. Serve immediately.

Nutrition: Calories: 253; Protein: 29g; Fiber: 4g; Fat: 16g; Carbs: 4g

Salmon and Sauce

Preparation Time: 25 minutes
Servings: 4
Ingredients:
4 salmon fillets; boneless
2 garlic cloves; minced
¼ cup ghee; melted
½ cup heavy cream
1 tbsp. chives; chopped.
1 tsp. lemon juice
1 tsp. dill; chopped.
A pinch of salt and black pepper
Directions:
Take a bowl and mix all the **Ingredients:** except the salmon and whisk well.
Arrange the salmon in a pan that fits the air fryer, drizzle the sauce all over, introduce the pan in the machine and cook at 360°F for 20 minutes. Divide everything between plates and serve
Nutrition: Calories: 220; Fat: 14g; Fiber: 2g; Carbs: 5g; Protein: 12g

Parmesan Cod

Preparation Time: 20 minutes
Servings: 4
Ingredients:
4 cod fillets; boneless
A drizzle of olive oil
3 spring onions; chopped.
1 cup parmesan
4 tbsp. balsamic vinegar
Salt and black pepper to taste.
Directions:
Season fish with salt, pepper, grease with the oil and coat it in parmesan.
Put the fillets in your air fryer's basket and cook at 370°F for 14 minutes. Meanwhile, in a bowl, mix the spring onions with salt, pepper and the vinegar and whisk
Divide the cod between plates, drizzle the spring onions mix all over and serve with a side salad
Nutrition: Calories: 220; Fat: 12g; Fiber: 2g; Carbs: 5g; Protein: 13g

Cod and Endives

Preparation Time: 25 minutes
Servings: 4
Ingredients:
4 salmon fillets; boneless
2 endives; shredded
2 tbsp. olive oil
½ tsp. sweet paprika
Salt and black pepper to the taste
Directions:
In a pan that fits the air fryer, combine the fish with the rest of the **Ingredients:**, toss, introduce in the fryer and cook at 350°F for 20 minutes, flipping the fish halfway
Divide between plates and serve right away
Nutrition: Calories: 243; Fat: 13g; Fiber: 3g; Carbs: 6g; Protein: 14g

Cod and Tomatoes

Preparation Time: 20 minutes
Servings: 4
Ingredients:
1 cup cherry tomatoes; halved
4 cod fillets, skinless and boneless
2 tbsp. olive oil
2 tbsp. cilantro; chopped.
Salt and black pepper to taste.
Directions:
In a baking dish that fits your air fryer, mix all the **Ingredients:**, toss gently.
Introduce in your air fryer and cook at 370°F for 15 minutes
Divide everything between plates and serve right away.
Nutrition: Calories: 248; Fat: 11g; Fiber: 2g; Carbs: 5g; Protein: 11g

Tarragon and Parmesan Trout

Preparation Time: 20 minutes
Servings: 4
Ingredients:
4 trout fillets; boneless
¾ cup parmesan; grated
2 garlic cloves; minced
½ cup chicken stock
¼ cup tarragon; chopped.
2 tbsp. olive oil
Salt and black pepper to taste.
Directions:
In a pan that fits your air fryer, mix all the **Ingredients:** except the fish and the parmesan and whisk. Add the fish and grease it well with this mix
Sprinkle the parmesan on top, put the pan in the air fryer and cook at 380°F for 15 minutes
Divide everything between plates and serve.
Nutrition: Calories: 271; Fat: 12g; Fiber: 4g; Carbs: 6g; Protein: 11g

Shrimp and Black Olives

Preparation Time: 17 minutes
Servings: 4
Ingredients:
1 lb. shrimp; peeled and deveined
1 tbsp. olive oil
4 garlic clove; minced
3 tbsp. parsley
1 cup black olives, pitted and chopped.
Directions:
In a pan that fits the air fryer, combine all the **Ingredients:**, toss.
Put the pan in the machine and cook at 380°F for 12 minutes. Divide between plates and serve
Nutrition: Calories: 251; Fat: 12g; Fiber: 3g; Carbs: 6g; Protein: 15g

Basil Cod

Preparation Time: 20 minutes
Servings: 4
Ingredients:
4 cod fillets; boneless
2 tbsp. olive oil
1 tsp. basil; dried
1 tsp. red pepper flakes
½ tsp. hot paprika
Salt and black pepper to taste.
Directions:
Take a bowl and mix the cod with all the other **Ingredients:** and toss.
Put the fish in your air fryer's basket and cook at 380°F for 15 minutes. Divide the cod between plates and serve
Nutrition: Calories: 194; Fat: 7g; Fiber: 2g; Carbs: 4g; Protein: 12g

Lime Baked Salmon

Preparation Time: 22 minutes
Servings: 2
Ingredients:
2 (3-oz.salmon fillets, skin removed
¼ cup sliced pickled jalapeños
½ medium lime, juiced
2 tbsp. chopped cilantro
1 tbsp. salted butter; melted.
½ tsp. finely minced garlic
1 tsp. chili powder
Directions:
Place salmon fillets into a 6-inch round baking pan. Brush each with butter and sprinkle with chili powder and garlic
Place jalapeño slices on top and around salmon. Pour half of the lime juice over the salmon and cover with foil. Place pan into the air fryer basket. Adjust the temperature to 370 Degrees F and set the timer for 12 minutes
When fully cooked, salmon should flake easily with a fork and reach an internal temperature of at least 145 Degrees F.
To serve, spritz with remaining lime juice and garnish with cilantro.
Nutrition: Calories: 167; Protein: 18g; Fiber: 7g; Fat: 9g; Carbs: 6g

Sea Bass and Fennel.

Preparation Time: 25 minutes
Servings: 2
Ingredients:
¼ cup black olives, pitted and sliced
2 sea bass, fillets
¼ cup basil; chopped.
1 fennel bulb; sliced
Juice of 1 lemon
1 tbsp. olive oil
A pinch of salt and black pepper

Directions:
In a pan that fits the air fryer, combine all the **Ingredients:**.
Introduce the pan in the machine and cook at 380°F for 20 minutes, shaking the fryer halfway.
Divide between plates and serve
Nutrition: Calories: 254; Fat: 10g; Fiber: 4g; Carbs: 6g; Protein: 11g

Snapper and Spring Onions

Preparation Time: 19 minutes
Servings: 4
Ingredients:
4 snapper fillets; boneless and skin scored
6 spring onions; chopped.
Juice of ½ lemon
3 tbsp. olive oil
2 tbsp. sweet paprika
A pinch of salt and black pepper
Directions:
Take a bowl and mix the paprika with the rest of the **Ingredients:** except the fish and whisk well
Rub the fish with this mix, place the fillets in your air fryer's basket and cook at 390°F for 7 minutes on each side.
Divide between plates and serve with a side salad.
Nutrition: Calories: 241; Fat: 12g; Fiber: 4g; Carbs: 6g; Protein: 13g

Herbed Trout and Asparagus

Preparation Time: 25 minutes
Servings: 4
Ingredients:
4 trout fillets; boneless and skinless
1 bunch asparagus; trimmed
¼ cup mixed chives and tarragon
2 tbsp. ghee; melted
2 tbsp. olive oil
1 tbsp. lemon juice
A pinch of salt and black pepper
Directions:
Mix the asparagus with half of the oil, salt and pepper, put it in your air fryer's basket, cook at 380°F for 6 minutes and divide between plates
Take a bowl and mix the trout with salt, pepper, lemon juice, the rest of the oil and the herbs and toss,
Put the fillets in your air fryer's basket and cook at 380°F for 7 minutes on each side
Divide the fish next to the asparagus, drizzle the melted ghee all over and serve
Nutrition: Calories: 240; Fat: 12g; Fiber: 4g; Carbs: 6g; Protein: 9g

Coco Shrimp

Preparation Time: 11 minutes
Servings: 2
Ingredients:
8 oz. medium shelled and deveined shrimp
¼ cup unsweetened shredded coconut
2 tbsp. salted butter; melted.

½ tsp. Old Bay seasoning
Directions:
Take a large bowl, toss the shrimp in butter and Old Bay seasoning
Place shredded coconut in bowl. Coat each piece of shrimp in the coconut and place into the air fryer basket.
Adjust the temperature to 400 Degrees F and set the timer for 6 minutes. Gently turn the shrimp halfway through the cooking time. Serve immediately.
Nutrition: Calories: 252; Protein: 19g; Fiber: 0g; Fat: 18g; Carbs: 8g

Shrimp and Zucchinis

Preparation Time: 20 minutes
Servings: 4
Ingredients:
1 lb. shrimp; peeled and deveined
2 zucchinis; cut into medium cubes
1 tbsp. lemon juice
1 tbsp. olive oil
1 tbsp. garlic; minced
A pinch of salt and black pepper
Directions:
In a pan that fits the air fryer, combine all the **Ingredients:**, toss, put the pan in the machine and cook at 370°F for 15 minutes.
Divide between plates and serve right away
Nutrition: Calories: 221; Fat: 9g; Fiber: 2g; Carbs: 15g; Protein: 11g

Trout and Zucchinis

Preparation Time: 20 minutes
Servings: 4
Ingredients:
3 zucchinis, cut in medium chunks
4 trout fillets; boneless
¼ cup tomato sauce
1 garlic clove; minced
½ cup cilantro; chopped.
1 tbsp. lemon juice
2 tbsp. olive oil
Salt and black pepper to taste.
Directions:
In a pan that fits your air fryer, mix the fish with the other **Ingredients:**, toss, introduce in the fryer and cook at 380°F for 15 minutes. Divide everything between plates and serve right away
Nutrition: Calories: 220; Fat: 12g; Fiber: 4g; Carbs: 6g; Protein: 9g

Flounder Fillets

Preparation Time: 25 minutes
Servings: 4
Ingredients:
4 flounder fillets; boneless
1 cup parmesan; grated
2 tbsp. olive oil
4 tbsp. butter; melted
A pinch of salt and black pepper

Directions:
Take a bowl and mix the parmesan with salt, pepper, butter and the oil and stir well.
Arrange the fish in a pan that fits the air fryer, spread the parmesan mix all over, introduce in the fryer and cook at 400°F for 20 minutes
Divide between plates and serve with a side salad.
Nutrition: Calories: 251; Fat: 14g; Fiber: 5g; Carbs: 6g; Protein: 12g

Garlic Lemon Shrimp

Preparation Time: 11 minutes
Servings: 2
Ingredients:
8 oz. medium shelled and deveined shrimp
1 medium lemon.
2 tbsp. unsalted butter; melted.
½ tsp. minced garlic
½ tsp. Old Bay seasoning
Directions:
Zest lemon and then cut in half. Place shrimp in a large bowl and squeeze juice from ½ lemon on top of them.
Add lemon zest to bowl along with remaining **Ingredients:**. Toss shrimp until fully coated
Pour bowl contents into 6-inch round baking dish. Place into the air fryer basket.
Adjust the temperature to 400 Degrees F and set the timer for 6 minutes. Shrimp will be bright pink when fully cooked. Serve warm with pan sauce.
Nutrition: Calories: 190; Protein: 14g; Fiber: 4g; Fat: 18g; Carbs: 9g

Salmon Pan

Preparation Time: 17 minutes
Servings: 4
Ingredients:
1 lb. salmon fillets, boneless, skinless and cubed
1 tbsp. sesame seeds, toasted
1 tbsp. chives; chopped.
2 tbsp. lime juice
1 tbsp. coconut aminos
1 tbsp. ginger; grated
4 tsp. olive oil
Directions:
In a pan that fits the air fryer, combine all the **Ingredients:**, toss.
Introduce in the fryer and cook at 360°F for 12 minutes. Divide into bowls and serve
Nutrition: Calories: 206; Fat: 8g; Fiber: 1g; Carbs: 4g; Protein: 13g

Buttery Cod

Preparation Time: 13 minutes
Servings: 2
Ingredients:
2 (4-oz.cod fillets
½ medium lemon, sliced
2 tbsp. salted butter; melted.
1 tsp. Old Bay seasoning

Directions:
Place cod fillets into a 6-inch round baking dish. Brush each fillet with butter and sprinkle with Old Bay seasoning. Lay two lemon slices on each fillet
Cover the dish with foil and place into the air fryer basket. Adjust the temperature to 350 Degrees F and set the timer for 8 minutes
Flip halfway through the cooking time. When cooked, internal temperature should be at least 145 Degrees F. Serve warm.
Nutrition: Calories: 179; Protein: 14g; Fiber: 0g; Fat: 11g; Carbs: 0g

Garlic Shrimp

Preparation Time: 17 minutes
Servings: 4
Ingredients:
1 lb. shrimp; peeled and deveined
4 garlic cloves; minced
1 tbsp. lime juice
2 tbsp. olive oil
2 tbsp. parsley; chopped.
1 tsp. cumin, ground
A pinch of salt and black pepper
Directions:
In a pan that fits your air fryer, mix all the **Ingredients:**, toss, put the pan in your air fryer and cook at 370°F and cook for 12 minutes, shaking the fryer halfway
Divide into bowls and serve.
Nutrition: Calories: 220; Fat: 11g; Fiber: 2g; Carbs: 5g; Protein: 12g

Spicy Peanut Butter Shrimp

Preparation Time: 15 minutes
Servings: 5
Ingredients:
1 ½ pound shrimp
Juice of 1 lemon
1 tsp sugar
3 tbsp peanut oil
2 tbsp cornstarch
2 scallions, chopped
¼ tsp Chinese powder
Chopped chili to taste
1 tsp salt
4 garlic cloves
1 tsp pepper
Directions:
Preheat the Air fryer to 370 F, and in a Ziploc bag, mix lemon juice, sugar, pepper, oil, cornstarch, powder, Chinese powder and salt. Add in the shrimp and massage to coat evenly. Let sit for 10 minutes.
Add garlic cloves, scallions and chili to a pan, and fry for a few minutes over medium heat. Place the marinated shrimp, garlic, chili and scallions in your air fryer's basket and cook for 10 minutes, until nice and crispy.

Crispy Calamari Rings

Preparation Time: 20 minutes
Servings: 5
Ingredients:
12 oz frozen squid
1 large egg, beaten
1 cup all-purpose flour
1 tsp ground coriander seeds
1 tsp cayenne pepper
½ tsp pepper
½ tsp salt
Lemon wedges, to garnish
olive oil for spray
Directions:
In a bowl, mix flour, ground pepper, paprika, cayenne pepper and salt. Dredge calamari in eggs, followed by the floured mixture. Preheat your Air Fryer to 390 F and cook them for 15 minutes, until golden brown. Do it in batches if needed to avoid overcrowding. Garnish with lemon wedges and enjoy!

Gingery Shrimp Medley

Preparation Time: 20 minutes
Servings: 4
Ingredients:
1 pound shrimp
2 whole onions, chopped
3 tbsp butter
1 ½ tbsp sugar
2 tbsp soy sauce
2 cloves garlic, chopped
2 tsp lime juice
1 tsp ginger, chopped
Directions:
Preheat your Air fryer to 340 F, and in a bowl, mix lime juice, soy sauce, ginger, garlic, sugar and butter.
Add the mixture to a frying pan and warm over medium heat. Add in the chopped onions, and cook for 1 minute until translucent. Pour the mixture over shrimp, toss well and set aside for 30 minutes. Then, place the mixture in the air fryer's basket and cook for 8 minutes.

Scrumptious Alaskan Salmon with Parsley Sauce

Preparation Time: 30 minutes
Servings: 4
Ingredients:
For Salmon
4 Alaskan wild salmon fillets, 6 oz each
2 tsp olive oil
A pinch of salt
For Dill Sauce
½ cup heavy cream
½ cup milk
A pinch of salt

2 tbsp chopped parsley
Directions:
Preheat your Air fryer to 310 F, and in a mixing bowl, add salmon and drizzle 1 tsp of oil. Season with salt and pepper. Place the salmon in your Air Fryer's cooking basket and cook for 20-25 minutes, until tender and crispy.
In a bowl, mix milk, chopped parsley, salt, and whipped cream. Serve the salmon with the sauce.

Creamy Onion Frittata with Smoked Trout

Preparation Time: 12 minutes
Servings: 6
Ingredients:
2 tbsp olive oil
1 onion, sliced
1 egg, beaten
6 tbsp crème fraiche
½ tbsp horseradish sauce
2 trout fillet, hot and smoked
A handful of fresh dill
Directions:
Heat oil in a frying pan over medium heat. Add onion and stir-fry until tender; season the onions well. Preheat your Air fryer to 320 F, and in a bowl, mix egg, crème Fraiche, and horseradish. Add cooked onion and trout, and mix well. Place the mixture in your fryer's cooking basket and cook for 20 minutes. Serve and enjoy!

Effortless Fish Nuggets with Garlic & Paprika

Preparation Time: 20 minutes
Servings: 4
Ingredients:
28 oz fish fillets
Lemon juice to taste
Salt and black pepper to taste
1 tsp drilled dill
4 tbsp mayonnaise
1 whole egg, beaten
1 tbsp garlic powder
3 ½ oz breadcrumbs
1 tbsp paprika
Directions:
Preheat your air fryer to 400 F, and season fish fillets with salt and pepper. In a bowl, mix beaten egg, lemon juice, and mayonnaise. In a separate bowl, mix breadcrumbs, paprika, dill, and garlic powder.
Dredge fillets in egg mixture and then the garlic-paprika mix; repeat until all fillets are prepared. Place the fillets in your Air Fryer's cooking basket and cook for 15 minutes. Serve and enjoy!

Lovely Cod Fillets with Fennel & Grapes

Preparation Time: 15 minutes
Servings: 4
Ingredients:
2 black cod fillets
Salt and black pepper to taste
1 cup grapes, halved

1 small fennel bulb, sliced
½ cup pecans
2 tsp white balsamic vinegar
2 tbsp extra virgin olive oil

Directions:

Preheat your Air fryer to 400 F, and season the fillets with salt and pepper; drizzle oil on top. Place the fillet in the air fryer basket and cook for 10 minutes; set the fish aside to cool. In a bowl, add grapes, pecans, and fennels. Drizzle oil over the grape mixture, and season with salt and pepper.

Add the mixture to the basket and cook for 3 minutes. Add balsamic vinegar and oil to the mixture, season with salt and pepper. Pour over the fish, and serve.

Parmesan Fish with Pine Nuts

Preparation Time: 15 minutes
Servings: 6
Ingredients:

1 Bunch of basil
2 garlic cloves, minced
1 tbsp olive oil
1 tbsp Parmesan cheese , grated
Black pepper and salt to taste
2 tbsp Pine nuts
6 white fish fillet
2 tbsp olive oil

Directions:

Season the fillets with salt and pepper. Preheat the Air fryer to 350 F, and cook the fillets inside for 8 minutes.

In a bowl, add basil, oil, pine nuts, garlic and Parmesan cheese; blend with your hand. Serve with the fish and enjoy!

Savory Cod Fish in Soy Sauce

Preparation Time: 20 minutes
Servings: 4
Ingredients:

7 ¼ oz codfish fillets
4 tbsp chopped cilantro
Salt to taste
A handful of green onions, chopped
1 cup water
5 slices of ginger
5 tbsp light soy sauce
3 tbsp oil
1 tsp dark soy sauce
5 cubes rock sugar

Directions:

Preheat your Air fryer to 360 F, and cover codfish with salt and coriander; drizzle with oil. Place the fish fillet in your air fryer's cooking basket and cook for 15 minutes. Place the remaining **Ingredients:** in a frying pan over medium heat; cook for 5 minutes. Serve the fish with the sauce, and enjoy.

Chili-Rubbed Jumbo Shrimp

Preparation Time: 10 minutes
Servings: 2 to 3
Ingredients:
1 lb jumbo shrimp
Salt to taste
¼ tsp old bay seasoning
⅓ tsp smoked paprika
¼ tsp chili powder
1 tbsp olive oil
Directions:
Preheat the Air fryer to 390 degrees. In a bowl, add the shrimp, paprika, oil, salt, old bay seasoning, and chili powder; mix well. Place the shrimp in the fryer, close and cook for 5 minutes. Serve with mayo and rice.

Delightful Catfish Fillets

Preparation Time: 25 minutes
Servings: 4
Ingredients:
4 catfish fillets, rinsed and dried
¼ cup seasoned fish fry
1 tbsp olive oil
1 tbsp parsley, chopped
Directions:
Preheat your Air fryer to 400 F, and add seasoned fish fry, and fillets in a large Ziploc bag; massage well to coat. Place the fillets in your Air fryer's cooking basket and cook for 10 minutes. Flip the fish and cook for 2-3 more minutes. Top with parsley and serve.

Shrimp with Smoked Paprika & Cayenne Pepper

Preparation Time: 10 minutes
Servings: 4
Ingredients:
5-6 oz tiger shrimp, 12 to 16 pieces
1 tbsp olive oil
½ a tbsp old bay seasoning
¼ a tbsp cayenne pepper
¼ a tbsp smoked paprika
A pinch of sea salt
Directions:
Preheat the Air fryer to 380 F, and mix all **Ingredients:** in a large bowl. Coat the shrimp with a little bit of oil and spices. Place the shrimp in the Air fryer's basket and fry for 6-7 minutes. Serve with rice or salad.

Speedy Fried Scallops

Preparation Time: 5 minutes
Servings: 6
Ingredients:
12 fresh scallops
3 tbsp flour
4 salt and black pepper
1 egg, lightly beaten

1 cup breadcrumbs

Directions:

Coat the scallops with flour. Dip into the egg, then into the breadcrumbs. Spray them with olive oil and arrange them in the air fryer. Cook for 6 minutes at 360 F, turning once halfway through cooking.

Simple Lemony Salmon

Preparation Time: 20 minutes

Servings: 2

Ingredients:

2 salmon fillets

Salt, to taste

Zest of a lemon

Directions:

Spray the fillets with olive oil and rub them with salt and lemon zest. Line baking paper in your air fryer's basket to avoid sticking. Cook the fillets for 10 minutes at 360 F, turning once halfway through. Serve with steamed asparagus and a drizzle of lemon juice.

Fried Cod Nuggets

Preparation Time: 25 minutes

Servings: 4

Ingredients:

1 ¼ lb cod fillets, cut into 4 to 6 chunks each

½ cup flour

1 egg

1 tbsp water

1 cup cornflakes

1 tbsp olive oil Salt and black pepper to taste

Directions:

Place the oil and cornflakes in a food processor and process until crumbed. Season the fish chunks with salt and pepper. In a bowl, beat the egg along with water. Dredge the chunks in flour first, then dip in the egg, and coat with cornflakes. Arrange on a lined sheet, and cook in the air fryer at 350 F for 15 minutes, until crispy.

Crispy Crab Legs

Preparation Time: 15 minutes

Servings: 3

Ingredients:

3 pounds crab legs

2 cups butter

1 cup salted water

Directions:

Preheat the Air fryer to 380 F, and dip the crab legs in salted water; let stay for a few minutes. Place the crab legs in the basket and cook for 10 minutes. Melt the butter in a bowl in the microwave. Pour over crab legs to serve.

Quick Shrimp Bowl

Preparation Time: 15 minutes

Servings: 6

Ingredients:

1 ¼ pound tiger shrimp

¼ tsp cayenne pepper
½ tsp old bay seasoning
¼ tsp smoked paprika
A pinch of salt
1 tbsp olive oil

Directions:

Preheat your Air fryer to 390 F, and in a bowl, mix all listed **Ingredients:**. Place the mixture in your air fryer's cooking basket and cook for 5 minutes. Serve with warm rice and a drizzle of lemon juice.

Garlic-Butter Catfish

Preparation Time: 20 minutes
Servings: 2
Ingredients:

2 catfish fillets
2 tsp blackening seasoning
Juice of 1 lime
2 tbsp butter, melted
1 garlic clove, mashed
2 tbsp cilantro

Directions:

Preheat your Air fryer to 360 degrees F, and in a bowl, blend in garlic, lime juice, cilantro and butter. Divide the sauce into two parts, pour 1 part of the sauce over your fillets; cover the fillets with seasoning.

Place the fillets in your Air fryer's basket and cook for 15 minutes. Serve the cooked fish with remaining sauce.

Delicious Fried Seafood

Preparation Time: 15 minutes
Servings: 4
Ingredients:

1 lb fresh scallops, mussels, fish fillets, prawns, shrimp
2 eggs, lightly beaten
Salt and black pepper
1 cup breadcrumbs mixed with the zest of 1 lemon

Directions:

Clean the seafood as needed. Dip each piece into the egg; and season with salt and pepper. Coat in the crumbs and spray with oil. Arrange into your air fryer and cook for 6 minutes at 400 F, turning once halfway through.

Easy Salmon Cakes

Preparation Time: 15 minutes
Servings: 2
Ingredients:

8 oz salmon, cooked
1 ½ oz potatoes, mashed
A handful of capers
A handful of parsley, chopped
Zest of 1 lemon
1 ¾ oz plain flour

Directions:
Carefully flake the salmon. In a bowl, mix flaked salmon, zest, capers, dill, and mashed potatoes. Form small cakes using the mixture and dust the cakes with flour; refrigerate for 60 minutes. Preheat your Air Fryer to 350 and cook the cakes for 7 minutes. Serve chilled.

Cheesy Tilapia Fillets

Preparation Time: 15 minutes
Servings: 4
Ingredients:
3/4 cup grated Parmesan cheese
1 tbsp olive oil
2 tsp paprika
1 tbsp chopped parsley
1/4 tsp garlic powder
1/4 tsp salt
4 tilapia fillets
Directions:
Preheat the Air fryer to 350 F, and mix parsley, Parmesan cheese, garlic, salt, and paprika in a shallow bowl. Brush the olive oil over the fillets, and then coat them with the Parmesan mixture. Place the tilapia onto a lined baking sheet, and then into the Air fryer. Cook for 4 to 5 minutes on all sides.

Rosemary Buttery Prawns

Preparation Time: 1 h 15 minutes
Servings: 2
Ingredients:
8 large prawns
3 garlic cloves, minced
1 rosemary sprig, chopped
1/2 tbsp melted butter
Salt and black pepper to taste
Directions:
Combine garlic, butter, rosemary, salt and pepper, in a bowl. Add the prawns to the bowl and mix to coat them well. Cover the bowl and refrigerate for an hour. Preheat the air fryer to 350 F, and cook for 6 minutes. Increase the temperature to 390 degrees, and cook for one more minute.

Old Bay Tilapia Fillets

Preparation Time: 15 minutes
Servings: 4
Ingredients:
1 pound tilapia fillets
1 tbsp old bay seasoning
2 tbsp canola oil
2 tbsp lemon pepper
Salt to taste
2-3 butter buds
Directions:
Preheat your Fryer to 400 F, and drizzle oil over tilapia fillet. In a bowl, mix salt, lemon pepper, butter buds, and seasoning; spread on the fish. Place the fillets in the Air fryer and cook for 10 minutes, until tender and crispy.

Sweet Cajun Salmon

Preparation Time: 10 minutes
Servings: 1
Ingredients:
1 salmon fillet
¼ tsp brown sugar
Juice of ½ lemon
1 tbsp cajun seasoning
2 lemon wedges
1 tbsp chopped parsley, for garnishing
Directions:
Preheat the Air fryer to 350 F, and combine sugar and lemon; coat the salmon with this mixture. Coat with the Cajun seasoning as well. Place a parchment paper into the air fryer and cook the fish for 7 minutes. Serve with lemon wedges and chopped parsley.

Lemon-Garlic Butter Lobster

Preparation Time: 15 minutes
Servings: 3
Ingredients:
4 oz lobster tails
1 tsp garlic, minced
1 tbsp butter
Salt and black pepper to taste
½ tbsp lemon Juice
Directions:
Add all the **Ingredients:** to a food processor, except shrimp, and blend well. Wash lobster and halve using meat knife; clean the skin of the lobster and cover the lobster with the marinade. Preheat your Air fryer to 380 F.
Place the lobster in your Air Fryer's cooking basket and cook for 10 minutes. Serve with fresh herbs and enjoy!

Shrimp and Arugula

Preparation Time: 3 minutes
Cooking time: 12 minutes
Servings: 4
Ingredients:
1 pound shrimp, peeled and deveined
1 cup baby arugula
A pinch of salt and black pepper
1 tablespoon parsley, chopped
½ teaspoon Italian seasoning
1 tablespoon olive oil
Directions:
In your air fryer, combine the shrimp with the arugula, oil and the other **Ingredients:**, toss and cook at 370 degrees F for 12 minutes.
Divide the shrimp mix into bowls and serve,
Nutrition: calories 199, fat 11, fiber 2, carbs 4, protein 11

BBQ Cod

Preparation Time: 5 minutes
Cooking time: 15 minutes
Servings: 4
Ingredients:
4 cod fillets, boneless
1 cup bbq sauce
1 cup baby spinach
1 teaspoon hot paprika
½ teaspoon oregano, dried
1 tablespoon avocado oil
Salt and black pepper to the taste
Directions:
In the air fryer's pan, combine the cod with the bbq sauce and the other **Ingredients:**, toss gently and cook at 380 degrees F for 15 minutes.
Divide the mix between plates and serve.
Nutrition: calories 194, fat 7, fiber 2, carbs 4, protein 12

Tuna and Shrimp Mix

Preparation Time: 5 minutes
Cooking time: 12 minutes
Servings: 4
Ingredients:
1 pound shrimp, peeled and deveined
½ pound tuna fillets, boneless and cubed
2 tablespoons olive oil
½ cup baby spinach
1 tablespoon lemon juice
1 cup cherry tomatoes, halved
4 garlic cloves, minced
Salt and black pepper to the taste
1 tablespoon chives, chopped
Directions:
In your air fryer, combine the shrimp with the tuna and the other **Ingredients:**, toss gently and cook at 380 degrees F for 12 minutes.
Divide into bowls and serve.
Nutrition: calories 220, fat 14, fiber 2, carbs 6, protein 15

Soy Sauce Cod

Preparation Time: 5 minutes
Cooking time: 16 minutes
Servings: 4
Ingredients:
4 cod fillets, boneless
3 tablespoons soy sauce
3 garlic cloves, minced
2 scallions, chopped
2 tablespoons olives oil
Salt and black pepper to the taste
2 tablespoons coriander, chopped

Directions:
In a bowl, combine the cod with the soy sauce, garlic and the other **Ingredients:**, rub well, transfer the fish to the air fryer's basket and cook at 370 degrees F for 16 minutes, flipping the fish halfway.
Divide between plates and serve with a side salad.
Nutrition: calories 270, fat 12, fiber 8, carbs 16, protein 14

Mackerel and Leeks

Preparation Time: 10 minutes
Cooking time: 15 minutes
Servings: 4
Ingredients:
4 mackerel fillets, boneless
2 garlic cloves, minced
1 tablespoon avocado oil
Salt and black pepper to the taste
2 leeks, sliced
2 tablespoons walnuts, chopped
1 tablespoon chives, chopped
Directions:
In your air fryer, combine the fish with the garlic, oil and the other **Ingredients:**, toss gently and cook at 360 degrees F for 15 minutes.
Divide the fish mix between plates and serve.
Nutrition: calories 280, fat 4, fiber 2, carbs 12, protein 15

VEGETARIAN

Balsamic Artichokes

Preparation Time: 10 minutes
Cooking duration: 7 minutes
Servings: 4
Ingredients:
4 big artichokes, trimmed
Salt and black pepper to the taste
2 tablespoons lemon juice
¼ cup extra virgin olive oil
2 teaspoons balsamic vinegar
1 teaspoon oregano, dried
2 garlic cloves, minced
Direction:
Spice artichokes with salt and pepper, rub them with half of the oil and half of the lemon juice, put them in your air fryer and cook at 360 °F for 7 minutes.
Meanwhile, in a bowl, mix the rest of the lemon juice with vinegar, the remaining oil, salt, pepper, garlic and oregano and stir very well.
Arrange artichokes on a platter, drizzle the balsamic vinaigrette over them and serve.

Cheesy Artichokes

Preparation Time: 10 minutes
Cooking duration: 6 minutes
Servings: 6
Ingredients:
14 ounces canned artichoke hearts
8 ounces cream cheese
16 ounces parmesan cheese, grated
10 ounces spinach
1/2 cup chicken stock
8 ounces mozzarella, shredded
1/2 cup sour cream
3 garlic cloves, minced
1/2 cup mayonnaise
1 teaspoon onion powder
Direction:
In a pan that fits your air fryer, mix artichokes with stock, garlic, spinach, cream cheese, sour cream, onion powder and mayo, toss, introduce in your air fryer and cook at 350 °F for 6 minutes.
Add mozzarella and parmesan, stir well and serve.

Artichokes and Special Sauce

Preparation Time: 10 minutes
Cooking duration: 6 minutes
Servings: 2
Ingredients:
2 artichokes, trimmed
A drizzle of olive oil
2 garlic cloves, minced
1 tablespoon lemon juice

For the sauce:
¼ cup coconut oil
¼ cup extra virgin olive oil
3 anchovy fillets
3 garlic cloves
Direction:
In a bowl, mix artichokes with oil, 2 garlic cloves and lemon juice, tosswell, transfer to your air fryer, cook at 350 °F for 6 minutes and divide among plates.
In your food processor, mix coconut oil with anchovy, 3 garlic cloves and olive oil, blend very well, drizzle over artichokes and serve.

Beet Salad and Parsley Dressing

Preparation Time: 10 minutes
Cooking duration: 14 minutes
Servings: 4
Ingredients:
4 beets
2 tablespoons balsamic vinegar
A bunch of parsley, diced
Salt and black pepper to the taste
1 tablespoon extra-virgin olive oil
1 garlic clove, diced
2 tablespoons capers
Direction:
Put beets in your air fryer and cook them at 360 °F for 14minutes.
Meanwhile, in a bowl, mix parsley with garlic, salt, pepper, olive oil and capers and stir very well.
Transfer beets to a cutting board, leave them to cool down, peel them, slice and put them in a salad bowl.
Add vinegar, drizzle the parsley dressing all over and serve.

Beets and Blue Cheese Salad

Preparation Time: 10 minutes
Cooking duration: 14 minutes
Servings: 6
Ingredients:
6 beets, peeled and quartered
Salt and black pepper to the taste
¼ cup blue cheese, crumbled
1 tablespoon olive oil
Direction:
Put beets in your air fryer, cook them at 350 °F for 14 minutes and transfer them to a bowl.
Add blue cheese, salt, pepper and oil, toss and serve.

Beet, Tomato and Goat Cheese Mix

Preparation Time: 30 minutes
Cooking duration: 14 minutes
Servings: 8
Ingredients:
8 small beets, trimmed, peeled and halved
1 red onion, sliced
4 ounces goat cheese, crumbled

1 tablespoon balsamic vinegar
Salt and black pepper to the taste
2 tablespoons sugar
1 pint mixed cherry tomatoes, halved
2 ounces pecans
2 tablespoons olive oil
Direction:
Put beets in your air fryer, spicethem with salt and pepper, cook at 350 °F for 14 minutes and transfer to a salad bowl.
Add onion, cherry tomatoes and pecans and toss.
In another bowl, mix vinegar with sugar and oil, whisk well until sugar dissolves and add to salad.
Also add goat cheese, toss and serve.

Broccoli Salad

Preparation Time: 10 minutes
Cooking duration: 8 minutes
Servings: 4
Ingredients:
1 broccoli head, florets separated
1 tablespoon peanut oil
6 garlic cloves, minced
1 tablespoon Chinese rice wine vinegar
Salt and black pepper to the taste
Direction:
In a bowl, mix broccoli with salt, pepper and half of the oil, toss, transfer to your air fryer and cook at 350 °F for 8 minutes, shaking the fryer halfway.
Transfer broccoli to a salad bowl, add the rest of the peanut oil, garlic and rice vinegar, toss really well and serve.

Brussels sprouts and Tomatoes Mix

Preparation Time: 5 minutes
Cooking duration: 10 minutes
Servings: 4
Ingredients:
1 pound Brussels sprouts, trimmed
Salt and black pepper to the taste
6 cherry tomatoes, halved
¼ cup green onions, diced
1 tablespoon olive oil
Direction:
Spice Brussels sprouts with salt and pepper, put them in your airfryer and cook at 350 °F for 10 minutes.
Transfer them to a bowl, add salt, pepper, cherry tomatoes, green onions and olive oil, toss well and serve.

Brussels sprouts and Butter Sauce.

Preparation Time: 4 minutes
Cooking duration: 10 minutes
Servings: 4
Ingredients:
1 pound Brussels sprouts, trimmed

Salt and black pepper to the taste
1/2 cup bacon, cooked and diced
1 tablespoon mustard
1 tablespoon butter
2 tablespoons dill, finely diced
Direction:
Put Brussels sprouts in your air fryer and cook them at 350 degrees
F for 10 minutes.
Heat up a pan with the butter over medium high heat, add bacon, mustard and dill and whisk well.
Divide Brussels sprouts on plates, drizzle butter sauce all over and serve.

Cheesy Brussels Sprouts

Preparation Time: 10 minutes
Cooking duration: 8 minutes
Servings: 4
Ingredients:
1 pound Brussels sprouts, washed
Juice of 1 lemon
Salt and black pepper to the taste
2 tablespoons butter
3 tablespoons parmesan, grated
Direction:
Put Brussels sprouts in your air fryer, cook them at 350 °Ffor 8 minutes and transfer them to a bowl.
Heat up a pan with the butter over medium heat, add lemon juice, salt and pepper, whisk well and add to Brussels sprouts.
Add parmesan, toss until parmesan melts and serve.

Spicy Cabbage

Preparation Time: 10 minutes
Cooking duration: 8 minutes
Servings: 4
Ingredients:
1 cabbage, cut into 8 wedges
1 tablespoon sesame seed oil
1 carrots, grated
¼ cup apple cider vinegar
¼ cups apple juice
1/2 teaspoon cayenne pepper
1 teaspoon red pepper flakes, crushed
Direction:
In a pan that fits your air fryer, combine cabbage with oil, carrot, vinegar, apple juice, cayenne and pepper flakes, introduce inpreheated air fryer and cook at 350 °F for 8 minutes.
Divide cabbage mix on plates and serve.

Sweet Baby Carrots Dish

Preparation Time: 10 minutes
Cooking duration: 10 minutes
Servings: 4
Ingredients:
2 cups baby carrots
A pinch of salt and black pepper
1 tablespoon brown sugar
1/2 tablespoon butter, melted
Direction:
In a dish that fits your air fryer, mix baby carrots with butter, salt, pepper and sugar, toss, introduce in your air fryer and cook at 350 °F for 10 minutes.
Divide among plates and serve.

Collard Greens and Turkey Wings

Preparation Time: 10 minutes
Cooking duration: 20 minutes
Servings: 6
Ingredients:
1 sweet onion, diced
2 smoked turkey wings
2 tablespoons olive oil
3 garlic cloves, minced
2 and 1/2 pounds collard greens, diced
Salt and black pepper to the taste
2 tablespoons apple cider vinegar
1 tablespoon brown sugar
1/2 teaspoon crushed red pepper
Direction:
Heat up a pan that fits your air fryer with the oil over medium high heat, add onions, stir and cook for 2 minutes.
Add garlic, greens, vinegar, salt, pepper, crushed red pepper, sugar and smoked turkey, introduce in preheated air fryer and cook at 350 °F for 15 minutes.
Divide greens and turkey on plates and serve.

Herbed Eggplant and Zucchini Mix

Preparation Time: 10 minutes
Cooking duration: 8 minutes
Servings: 4
Ingredients:
1 eggplant, roughly cubed
3 zucchinis, roughly cubed
2 tablespoons lemon juice
Salt and black pepper to the taste
1 teaspoon thyme, dried
1 teaspoon oregano, dried
3 tablespoons olive oil
Direction:
Put eggplant in a dish that fits your air fryer, add zucchinis, lemon juice, salt, pepper, thyme, oregano and olive oil, toss, introduce in your air fryer and cook at 360 °F for 8 minutes.

Divide among plates and serve right away.

Flavored Fennel

Preparation Time: 10 minutes
Cooking duration: 8 minutes
Servings: 4
Ingredients:
2 fennel bulbs, cut into quarters
3 tablespoons olive oil
Salt and black pepper to the taste
1 garlic clove, minced
1 red chili pepper, diced
¾ cup veggie stock
Juice from 1/2 lemon
¼ cup white wine
¼ cup parmesan, grated
Direction:
Heat up a pan that fits your air fryer with the oil over medium high heat, add garlic and chili pepper, stir and cook for 2 minutes.
Add fennel, salt, pepper, stock, wine, lemon juice, and parmesan, toss to coat, introduce in your air fryer and cook at 350 °Ffor 6 minutes.
Divide among plates and serve right away.

Crispy Potatoes and Parsley

Preparation Time: 10 minutes
Cooking time: 10 minutes
Servings:4
Ingredients:
1 pound gold potatoes, cut into wedges
Salt and black pepper to the taste
2 tablespoons olive
Juice from ½ lemon
¼ cup parsley leaves, chopped
Direction:
Rub potatoes with salt, pepper, lemon juice and olive oil, put them in your air fryer and cook at 350°F for 10 minutes.
Divide among plates, sprinkle parsley on top and serve.

Indian Turnips Salad

Preparation Time: 10 minutes
Cooking time: 12 minutes
Servings:4
Ingredients:
20 ounces turnips, peeled and chopped
1 teaspoon garlic, minced
1 teaspoon ginger, grated
2 yellow onions, chopped
2 tomatoes, chopped
1 teaspoon cumin, ground
1 teaspoon coriander, ground
2 green chilies, chopped

½ teaspoon turmeric powder
2 tablespoons butter
Salt and black pepper to the taste
A handful coriander leaves, chopped
Direction:
•Heat up a pan that fits your air fryer with the butter, melt it, add green chilies, garlic and ginger, stir and cook for 1 minute.
•Add onions, salt, pepper, tomatoes, turmeric, cumin, ground coriander and turnips, stir, introduce in your air fryer and cook at 350 °F for 10 minutes.
•Divide among plates, sprinkle fresh coriander on top and serve.

Simple Stuffed Tomatoes

Preparation Time: 10 minutes
Cooking duration: 15 minutes
Servings: 4
Ingredients:
4 tomatoes, tops cut off and pulp scooped and chopped Salt and black pepper to the taste
1 yellow onion, chopped
1 tablespoon butter
2 tablespoons celery, chopped
½ cup mushrooms, chopped
1 tablespoon bread crumbs
1 cup cottage cheese
¼ teaspoon caraway seeds
1 tablespoon parsley, chopped
Direction:
Heat up a pan with the butter over medium heat, melt it, add onion and celery, stir and cook for 3 minutes.
Add tomato pulp and mushrooms, stir and cook for 1 minute more.
Add salt, pepper, crumbled bread, cheese, caraway seeds and parsley, stir, cook for 4 minutes more and take off heat.
Stuff tomatoes with this mix, place them in your air fryer and cook at 350 °F for 8 minutes.
Divide stuffed tomatoes on plates and serve.

Indian Potatoes

Preparation Time: 10 minutes
Cooking duration: 12 minutes
Servings: 4
Ingredients:
1 tablespoon coriander seeds
1 tablespoon cumin seeds
Salt and black pepper to the taste
½ teaspoon turmeric powder
½ teaspoon red chili powder
1 teaspoon pomegranate powder
1 tablespoon pickled mango, chopped
2 teaspoons fenugreek, dried
5 potatoes, boiled, peeled and cubed
2 tablespoons olive oil
Direction:

Heat up a pan that fits your air fryer with the oil over medium heat, add coriander and cumin seeds, stir and cook for 2 minutes.
Add salt, pepper, turmeric, chili powder, pomegranate powder, mango, fenugreek and potatoes, toss, introduce in your air fryer and cook at 360 °F for 10 minutes.
Divide among plates and serve hot.

Broccoli and Tomatoes Air Fried Stew

Preparation Time: 10 minutes
Cooking duration: 20 minutes
Servings: 4
Ingredients:
1 broccoli head, florets separated
2 teaspoons coriander seeds
1 tablespoon olive oil
1 yellow onion, chopped
Salt and black pepper to the taste
A pinch of red pepper, crushed
1 small ginger piece, chopped
1 garlic clove, minced
28 ounces canned tomatoes, pureed
Direction:
Heat up a pan that fits your air fryer with the oil over medium heat, add onions, salt, pepper and red pepper, stir and cook for 7 minutes.
Add ginger, garlic, coriander seeds, tomatoes and broccoli, stir, introduce in your air fryer and cook at 360 °F for 12 minutes.
Divide into bowls and serve.

Sesame Mustard Greens

Preparation Time: 10 minutes
Cooking duration: 11 minutes
Servings: 4
Ingredients:
2 garlic cloves, minced
1 pound mustard greens, torn
1 tablespoon olive oil
½ cup yellow onion, sliced
Salt and black pepper to the taste
3 tablespoons veggie stock
¼ teaspoon dark sesame oil
Direction:
Heat up a pan that fits your air fryer with the oil over medium heat, add onions, stir and brown them for 5 minutes.
Add garlic, stock, greens, salt and pepper, stir, introduce in your air fryer and cook at 350 °F for 6 minutes.
Add sesame oil, toss to coat, divide among plates and serve.

Kale and Brussels Sprouts

Preparation Time: 20 minutes
Servings: 8
Ingredients:
1 lb. Brussels sprouts, trimmed

3 oz. mozzarella, shredded
2 cups kale, torn
1 tbsp. olive oil
Salt and black pepper to taste.
Directions:
In a pan that fits the air fryer, combine all the **Ingredients:** except the mozzarella and toss.
Put the pan in the air fryer and cook at 380°F for 15 minutes
Divide between plates, sprinkle the cheese on top and serve.
Nutrition: Calories: 170; Fat: 5g; Fiber: 3g; Carbs: 4g; Protein: 7g

Broccoli And Tomato Sauce

Preparation Time: 20 minutes
Servings: 4
Ingredients:
1 broccoli head, florets separated
¼ cup scallions; chopped
½ cup tomato sauce
1 tbsp. olive oil
1 tbsp. sweet paprika
Salt and black pepper to taste.
Directions:
In a pan that fits the air fryer, combine the broccoli with the rest of the **Ingredients:**, toss.
Put the pan in the fryer and cook at 380°F for 15 minutes
Divide between plates and serve.
Nutrition: Calories: 163; Fat: 5g; Fiber: 2g; Carbs: 4g; Protein: 8g

Kale and Olives

Preparation Time: 20 minutes
Servings: 4
Ingredients:
1 an ½ lb. kale, torn
1 tbsp. hot paprika
2 tbsp. olive oil
2 tbsp. black olives, pitted and sliced
Salt and black pepper to taste.
Directions:
In a pan that fits the air fryer, combine all the **Ingredients:** and toss.
Put the pan in your air fryer, cook at 370°F for 15 minutes, divide between plates and serve
Nutrition: Calories: 154; Fat: 3g; Fiber: 2g; Carbs: 4g; Protein: 6g

Zucchini and Olives

Preparation Time: 17 minutes
Servings: 4
Ingredients:
4 zucchinis; sliced
2 tbsp. olive oil
1 cup kalamata olives, pitted
2 tbsp. lime juice
2 tsp. balsamic vinegar
Salt and black pepper to taste.

Directions:
In a pan that fits your air fryer, mix the olives with all the other **Ingredients:**, toss, introduce in the fryer and cook at 390°F for 12 minutes
Divide the mix between plates and serve.
Nutrition: Calories: 150; Fat: 4g; Fiber: 2g; Carbs: 4g; Protein: 5g

Italian Olives

Preparation Time: 20 minutes
Servings: 4
Ingredients:
12 oz. tomatoes; chopped.
2 cups black olives, pitted and halved
4 garlic cloves; minced
2 rosemary springs; chopped.
2 red bell peppers; sliced
A handful basil; chopped.
2 tbsp. olive oil
Directions:
In a pan that fits the air fryer, combine the olives with the rest of the **Ingredients:**, toss.
Put the pan in the fryer and cook at 380°F for 15 minutes
Divide between plates and serve.
Nutrition: Calories: 173; Fat: 6g; Fiber: 2g; Carbs: 4g; Protein: 5g

Creamy Kale

Preparation Time: 20 minutes
Servings: 4
Ingredients:
2 lb. kale, torn
2 garlic cloves; minced
½ cup parmesan, grated
1 ½ cups coconut cream
2 tbsp. olive oil
½ tsp. nutmeg, ground
A pinch of salt and black pepper
Directions:
In a pan that fits your air fryer, mix the kale with the rest of the **Ingredients:**, toss, introduce the pan in the fryer and cook at 400°F for 15 minutes. Divide between plates and serve
Nutrition: Calories: 135; Fat: 3g; Fiber: 2g; Carbs: 4g; Protein: 6g

Broccoli Casserole

Preparation Time: 35 minutes
Servings: 4
Ingredients:
1 lb. broccoli florets
15 oz. coconut cream
2 eggs, whisked
2 cups cheddar, grated
1 cup parmesan, grated
1 tbsp. parsley; chopped
3 tbsp. ghee; melted
1 tbsp. mustard

A pinch of salt and black pepper

Directions:

Grease a baking pan that fits the air fryer with the ghee and arrange the broccoli on the bottom.

Add the cream, mustard, salt, pepper and the eggs and toss

Sprinkle the cheese on top, put the pan in the air fryer and cook at 380°F for 30 minutes

Divide between plates and serve.

Nutrition: Calories: 244; Fat: 12g; Fiber: 3g; Carbs: 5g; Protein: 12g

Broccoli and Almonds

Preparation Time: 17 minutes

Servings: 4

Ingredients:

1 lb. broccoli florets
½ cup almonds; chopped
3 garlic cloves; minced
1 tbsp. chives; chopped
2 tbsp. red vinegar
3 tbsp. coconut oil; melted
A pinch of salt and black pepper

Directions:

Take a bowl and mix the broccoli with the garlic, salt, pepper, vinegar and the oil and toss.

Put the broccoli in your air fryer's basket and cook at 380°F for 12 minutes

Divide between plates and serve with almonds and chives sprinkled on top.

Nutrition: Calories: 180; Fat: 4g; Fiber: 2g; Carbs: 4g; Protein: 6g

Oregano Kale

Preparation Time: 15 minutes

Servings: 4

Ingredients:

1 lb. kale, torn
2 tbsp. oregano; chopped
1 tbsp. olive oil
A pinch of salt and black pepper

Directions:

In a pan that fits the air fryer, combine all the **Ingredients:** and toss.

Put the pan in the air fryer and cook at 380°F for 10 minutes. Divide between plates and serve

Nutrition: Calories: 140; Fat: 3g; Fiber: 2g; Carbs: 3g; Protein: 5g

Italian Asparagus

Preparation Time: 15 minutes

Servings: 4

Ingredients:

1 lb. asparagus, trimmed
2 cups cherry tomatoes; halved
2 cups mozzarella, shredded
½ cup balsamic vinegar
2 tbsp. olive oil
A pinch of salt and black pepper

Directions:

In a pan that fits your air fryer, mix the asparagus with the rest of the **Ingredients:** except the mozzarella and toss

Put the pan in the air fryer and cook at 400°F for 10 minutes. Divide between plates and serve
Nutrition: Calories: 200; Fat: 6g; Fiber: 2g; Carbs: 3g; Protein: 6g

Lemon Endives

Preparation Time: 20 minutes
Servings: 4
Ingredients:
12 endives, trimmed
3 tbsp. ghee; melted
1 tbsp. lemon juice
A pinch of salt and black pepper
Directions:
Take a bowl and mix the endives with the ghee, salt, pepper and lemon juice and toss.
Put the endives in the fryer's basket and cook at 350°F for 15 minutes
Divide between plates and serve.
Nutrition: Calories: 163; Fat: 4g; Fiber: 3g; Carbs: 5g; Protein: 6g

Vinegar Broccoli

Preparation Time: 30 minutes
Servings: 4
Ingredients:
6 bacon slices, cooked and crumbled
1 broccoli head, florets separated
½ cup cranberries
½ cup almonds; chopped
2 shallots; chopped
3 tbsp. balsamic vinegar
A pinch of salt and black pepper
Directions:
In a pan that fits the air fryer, combine the broccoli with the rest of the **Ingredients:** and toss.
Put the pan in the air fryer and cook at 380°F for 25 minutes
Divide between plates and serve.
Nutrition: Calories: 173; Fat: 7g; Fiber: 2g; Carbs: 4g; Protein: 8g

Balsamic Kale

Preparation Time: 14 minutes
Servings: 6
Ingredients:
2 ½ lb. kale leaves
3 garlic cloves; minced
2 tbsp. olive oil
2 tbsp. balsamic vinegar
Salt and black pepper to taste.
Directions:
In a pan that fits the air fryer, combine all the **Ingredients:** and toss.
Put the pan in your air fryer and cook at 300°F for 12 minutes. Divide between plates and serve
Nutrition: Calories: 122; Fat: 4g; Fiber: 3g; Carbs: 4g; Protein: 5g

Kale and Mushrooms

Preparation Time: 20 minutes
Servings: 4
Ingredients:
1 lb. brown mushrooms; sliced
1 lb. kale, torn
14 oz. coconut milk
2 tbsp. olive oil
Salt and black pepper to taste.
Directions:
In a pan that fits your air fryer, mix the kale with the rest of the **Ingredients:** and toss
Put the pan in the fryer, cook at 380°F for 15 minutes, divide between plates and serve
Nutrition: Calories: 162; Fat: 4g; Fiber: 1g; Carbs: 3g; Protein: 5g

Mustard Asparagus

Preparation Time: 17 minutes
Servings: 4
Ingredients:
1 lb. asparagus, trimmed
½ cup parmesan, grated
¼ cup mustard
3 garlic cloves; minced
2 tbsp. olive oil
Directions:
Take a bowl and mix the asparagus with the oil, garlic and mustard and toss really well.
Put the asparagus spears in your air fryer's basket and cook at 400°F for 12 minutes
Divide between plates, sprinkle the parmesan on top and serve.
Nutrition: Calories: 162; Fat: 4g; Fiber: 4g; Carbs: 6g; Protein: 9g

Cajun Olives and Peppers

Preparation Time: 16 minutes
Servings: 4
Ingredients:
½ lb. mixed bell peppers; sliced
1 cup black olives, pitted and halved
½ tbsp. Cajun seasoning
1 tbsp. olive oil
Directions:
In a pan that fits the air fryer, combine all the **Ingredients:**.
Put the pan it in your air fryer and cook at 390°F for 12 minutes. Divide the mix between plates and serve
Nutrition: Calories: 151; Fat: 3g; Fiber: 2g; Carbs: 4g; Protein: 5g

Roasted Lemon Cauliflower

Preparation Time: 20 minutes
Servings: 4
Ingredients:
1 medium head cauliflower
1 medium lemon.
2 tbsp. salted butter; melted.
1 tsp. dried parsley.

½ tsp. garlic powder.

Directions:

Remove the leaves from the head of cauliflower and brush it with melted butter. Cut the lemon in half and zest one half onto the cauliflower. Squeeze the juice of the zested lemon half and pour it over the cauliflower.

Sprinkle with garlic powder and parsley. Place cauliflower head into the air fryer basket. Adjust the temperature to 350 Degrees F and set the timer for 15 minutes

Check cauliflower every 5 minutes to avoid overcooking. It should be fork tender.

To serve, squeeze juice from other lemon half over cauliflower. Serve immediately.

Nutrition: Calories: 91; Protein: 0g; Fiber: 2g; Fat: 7g; Carbs: 4g

Turmeric Cabbage

Preparation Time: 20 minutes

Servings: 4

Ingredients:

1 green cabbage head, shredded

¼ cup ghee; melted

1 tbsp. dill; chopped.

2 tsp. turmeric powder

Directions:

In a pan that fits your air fryer, mix the cabbage with the rest of the **Ingredients:** except the dill, toss, put the pan in the fryer and cook at 370°F for 15 minutes

Divide everything between plates and serve with dill sprinkled on top.

Nutrition: Calories: 173; Fat: 5g; Fiber: 3g; Carbs: 6g; Protein: 7g

Asparagus and Yogurt Sauce

Preparation Time: 14 minutes

Servings: 4

Ingredients:

1 lb. asparagus, trimmed

2 garlic cloves; minced

¼ cup chives; chopped

¼ cup lemon juice

1 cup Greek yogurt

1 cup basil; chopped

½ cup parsley; chopped

2 tbsp. olive oil

1 tsp. garlic powder

1 tsp. oregano; dried

A pinch of salt and black pepper

Directions:

Take a bowl and mix the asparagus with the oil, salt, pepper, oregano and garlic powder and toss.

Put the asparagus in the air fryer's basket and cook at 400°F for 10 minutes

Meanwhile, in a blender, mix the yogurt with basil, chives, parsley, lemon juice and garlic cloves and pulse well

Divide the asparagus between plates, drizzle the sauce all over and serve.

Nutrition: Calories: 194; Fat: 6g; Fiber: 2g; Carbs: 4g; Protein: 8g

Butter Broccoli

Preparation Time: 20 minutes
Servings: 4
Ingredients:
1 lb. broccoli florets
½ tbsp. butter; melted
1 tsp. sweet paprika
A pinch of salt and black pepper
Directions:
Take a bowl and mix the broccoli with the rest of the **Ingredients:** and toss.
Put the broccoli in your air fryer's basket, cook at 350°F for 15 minutes, divide between plates and serve
Nutrition: Calories: 130; Fat: 3g; Fiber: 3g; Carbs: 4g; Protein: 8g

Spicy Olives and Avocado

Preparation Time: 20 minutes
Servings: 4
Ingredients:
2 small avocados, pitted; peeled and sliced
¼ cup cherry tomatoes; halved
2 cups kalamata olives, pitted
1 tbsp. coconut oil; melted
Juice of 1 lime
Directions:
In a pan that fits the air fryer, combine the olives with the other **Ingredients:**, toss.
Put the pan in your air fryer and cook at 370°F for 15 minutes
Divide the mix between plates and serve.
Nutrition: Calories: 153; Fat: 3g; Fiber: 3g; Carbs: 4g; Protein: 6g

Roasted Asparagus

Preparation Time: 15 minutes
Servings: 4
Ingredients:
1 lb. asparagus, trimmed
1 tbsp. sweet paprika
3 tbsp. olive oil
A pinch of salt and black pepper
Directions:
Take a bowl and mix the asparagus with the rest of the **Ingredients:** and toss
Put the asparagus in your air fryer's basket and cook at 400°F for 10 minutes. Divide between plates and serve
Nutrition: Calories: 200; Fat: 5g; Fiber: 2g; Carbs: 4g; Protein: 6g

Parmesan Broccoli and Asparagus

Preparation Time: 20 minutes
Servings: 4
Ingredients:
½ lb. asparagus, trimmed
1 broccoli head, florets separated
Juice of 1 lime
3 tbsp. parmesan, grated

2 tbsp. olive oil
Salt and black pepper to taste.

Directions:

Take a bowl and mix the asparagus with the broccoli and all the other **Ingredients:** except the parmesan, toss, transfer to your air fryer's basket and cook at 400°F for 15 minutes

Divide between plates, sprinkle the parmesan on top and serve.

Nutrition: Calories: 172; Fat: 5g; Fiber: 2g; Carbs: 4g; Protein: 9g

Cauliflower Pizza Crust

Preparation Time: 26 minutes
Servings: 2
Ingredients:

1 (12-oz.steamer bag cauliflower
1 large egg.
½ cup shredded sharp Cheddar cheese.
2 tbsp. blanched finely ground almond flour
1 tsp. Italian blend seasoning

Directions:

Cook cauliflower according to package instructions. Remove from bag and place into cheesecloth or paper towel to remove excess water. Place cauliflower into a large bowl.

Add cheese, egg, almond flour and Italian seasoning to the bowl and mix well

Cut a piece of parchment to fit your air fryer basket. Press cauliflower into 6-inch round circle. Place into the air fryer basket. Adjust the temperature to 360 Degrees F and set the timer for 11 minutes. After 7 minutes, flip the pizza crust

Add preferred toppings to pizza. Place back into air fryer basket and cook an additional 4 minutes or until fully cooked and golden. Serve immediately.

Nutrition: Calories: 230; Protein: 19g; Fiber: 7g; Fat: 12g; Carbs: 10g

Tomato and Kale Salad

Preparation Time: 20 minutes
Servings: 4
Ingredients:

½ lb. kale leaves, torn
¼ cup veggie stock
10 cherry tomatoes; halved
2 tbsp. tomato sauce
Salt and black pepper to taste.

Directions:

In a pan that fits your air fryer, mix tomatoes with the remaining **Ingredients:**, toss.

Put the pan in the fryer and cook at 360°F for 15 minutes

Divide between plates and serve right away.

Nutrition: Calories: 161; Fat: 2g; Fiber: 2g; Carbs: 4g; Protein: 6g

Lemon Asparagus

Preparation Time: 17 minutes
Servings: 4
Ingredients:

1 lb. asparagus, trimmed
3 garlic cloves; minced
3 tbsp. parmesan, grated
2 tbsp. olive oil

Juice of 1 lemon
A pinch of salt and black pepper
Directions:
Take a bowl and mix the asparagus with the rest of the **Ingredients:** and toss.
Put the asparagus in your air fryer's basket and cook at 390°F for 12 minutes. Divide between plates and serve
Nutrition: Calories: 175; Fat: 5g; Fiber: 2g; Carbs: 4g; Protein: 8g

Veggie Quesadilla

Preparation Time: 15 minutes
Servings: 2
Ingredients:
4 flatbread dough tortillas
⅔ cup shredded pepper jack cheese
½ medium avocado; peeled, pitted and mashed
½ medium green bell pepper; seeded and chopped
¼ cup diced red onion
¼ cup chopped white mushrooms
¼ cup full-fat sour cream.
¼ cup mild salsa
1 tbsp. coconut oil
Directions:
In a medium skillet over medium heat, warm coconut oil. Add pepper, onion and mushrooms to skillet and sauté until peppers begin to soften, 3–5 minutes
Place two tortillas on a work surface and sprinkle each with half of cheese. Top with sautéed veggies, sprinkle with remaining cheese and place remaining two tortillas on top
Place quesadillas carefully into the air fryer basket.
Adjust the temperature to 400 Degrees F and set the timer for 5 minutes.
Flip the quesadillas halfway through the cooking time. Serve warm with avocado, sour cream and salsa.
Nutrition: Calories: 795; Protein: 35g; Fiber: 5g; Fat: 63g; Carbs: 14g

Chili Broccoli

Preparation Time: 20 minutes
Servings: 4
Ingredients:
1 lb. broccoli florets
Juice of 1 lime
2 tbsp. chili sauce
2 tbsp. olive oil
A pinch of salt and black pepper
Directions:
Take a bowl and mix the broccoli with the other **Ingredients:** and toss well.
Put the broccoli in your air fryer's basket and cook at 400°F for 15 minutes
Divide between plates and serve.
Nutrition: Calories: 173; Fat: 6g; Fiber: 2g; Carbs: 6g; Protein: 8g

Olives and Cilantro Vinaigrette

Preparation Time: 17 minutes
Servings: 4
Ingredients:
1 cup baby spinach
2 cups black olives, pitted
1 tbsp. olive oil
2 tbsp. balsamic vinegar
A bunch of cilantro; chopped.
Salt and black pepper to taste.
Directions:
In a pan that fits the air fryer, combine all the **Ingredients:** and toss.
Put the pan in the air fryer and cook at 370°F for 12 minutes
Transfer to bowls and serve.
Nutrition: Calories: 132; Fat: 4g; Fiber: 2g; Carbs: 4g; Protein: 4g

Parmesan Artichokes

Preparation Time: 20 minutes
Servings: 4
Ingredients:
¼ cup blanched finely ground almond flour.
2 medium artichokes, trimmed and quartered, center removed
1 large egg, beaten
½ cup grated vegetarian Parmesan cheese.
2 tbsp. coconut oil
½ tsp. crushed red pepper flakes.
Directions:
Take a large bowl, toss artichokes in coconut oil and then dip each piece into the egg.
Mix the Parmesan and almond flour in a large bowl. Add artichoke pieces and toss to cover as completely as possible, sprinkle with pepper flakes. Place into the air fryer basket
Adjust the temperature to 400 Degrees F and set the timer for 10 minutes. Toss the basket two times during cooking. Serve warm.
Nutrition: Calories: 189; Protein: 9g; Fiber: 2g; Fat: 15g; Carbs: 10g

Bacon Asparagus

Preparation Time: 15 minutes
Servings: 4
Ingredients:
2 lb. asparagus, trimmed
4 bacon slices, cooked and crumbled
1 cup cheddar cheese, shredded
4 garlic cloves; minced
2 tbsp. olive oil
Directions:
Take a bowl and mix the asparagus with the other **Ingredients:** except the bacon, toss and put in your air fryer's basket
Cook at 400°F for 10 minutes, divide between plates, sprinkle the bacon on top and serve.
Nutrition: Calories: 172; Fat: 6g; Fiber: 2g; Carbs: 5g; Protein: 8g

Garlic Tomatoes

Preparation Time: 20 minutes
Servings: 4
Ingredients:
1 lb. cherry tomatoes; halved
6 garlic cloves; minced
1 tbsp. olive oil
1 tbsp. dill; chopped.
1 tbsp. balsamic vinegar
Salt and black pepper to taste.
Directions:
In a pan that fits the air fryer, combine all the **Ingredients:**, toss gently.
Put the pan in the air fryer and cook at 380°F for 15 minutes
Divide between plates and serve.
Nutrition: Calories: 121; Fat: 3g; Fiber: 2g; Carbs: 4g; Protein: 6g

Fennel and Collard Greens Sauté

Preparation Time: 17 minutes
Servings: 4
Ingredients:
1 lb. collard greens, trimmed
½ cup tomato sauce
2 fennel bulbs, trimmed and quartered
2 tbsp. olive oil
Salt and black pepper to taste.
Directions:
In a pan that fits your air fryer, mix the collard greens with the fennel and the rest of the **Ingredients:**, toss, put the pan in the fryer and cook at 350°F for 12 minutes
Divide everything between plates and serve.
Nutrition: Calories: 163; Fat: 4g; Fiber: 3g; Carbs: 5g; Protein: 6g

Olives and Artichokes

Preparation Time: 20 minutes
Servings: 4
Ingredients:
14 oz. canned artichoke hearts, drained
½ cup tomato sauce
2 cups black olives, pitted
3 garlic cloves; minced
1 tbsp. olive oil
1 tsp. garlic powder
Directions:
In a pan that fits your air fryer, mix the olives with the artichokes and the other **Ingredients:**, toss, put the pan in the fryer and cook at 350°F for 15 minutes
Divide the mix between plates and serve.
Nutrition: Calories: 180; Fat: 4g; Fiber: 3g; Carbs: 5g; Protein: 6g

Spinach Cheese Pie

Preparation Time: 30 minutes
Servings: 4
Ingredients:
1 cup frozen chopped spinach, drained
¼ cup heavy whipping cream.
1 cup shredded sharp Cheddar cheese.
¼ cup diced yellow onion
6 large eggs.
Directions:
Take a medium bowl, whisk eggs and add cream. Add remaining **Ingredients:** to bowl.
Pour into a 6-inch round baking dish. Place into the air fryer basket. Adjust the temperature to 320 Degrees F and set the timer for 20 minutes
Eggs will be firm and slightly browned when cooked. Serve immediately.
Nutrition: Calories: 288; Protein: 10g; Fiber: 3g; Fat: 20g; Carbs: 9g

Savoy Cabbage and Tomatoes

Preparation Time: 20 minutes
Servings: 4
Ingredients:
2 spring onions; chopped.
1 savoy cabbage, shredded
1 tbsp. parsley; chopped.
2 tbsp. tomato sauce
Salt and black pepper to taste.
Directions:
In a pan that fits your air fryer, mix the cabbage the rest of the **Ingredients:** except the parsley, toss, put the pan in the fryer and cook at 360°F for 15 minutes
Divide between plates and serve with parsley sprinkled on top.
Nutrition: Calories: 163; Fat: 4g; Fiber: 3g; Carbs: 6g; Protein: 7g

Kale and Bell Peppers

Preparation Time: 15 minutes
Servings: 4
Ingredients:
1 ½ cups avocado, peeled, pitted and cubed
2 cups kale, torn
¼ cup olive oil
1 cup red bell pepper; sliced
1 tbsp. white vinegar
2 tbsp. lime juice
1 tbsp. mustard
A pinch of salt and black pepper
Directions:
In a pan that fits the air fryer, combine the kale with salt, pepper, avocado and half of the oil, toss.
Put in your air fryer and cook at 360°F for 10 minutes
In a bowl, combine the kale mix with the rest of the **Ingredients:**, toss and serve.
Nutrition: Calories: 131; Fat: 3g; Fiber: 2g; Carbs: 4g; Protein: 5g

Broccoli and Tomatoes

Preparation Time: 20 minutes
Servings: 4
Ingredients:
1 broccoli head, florets separated
2 cups cherry tomatoes, quartered
1 tbsp. cilantro; chopped.
Juice of 1 lime
A drizzle of olive oil
A pinch of salt and black pepper
Directions:
In a pan that fits the air fryer, combine the broccoli with tomatoes and the rest of the **Ingredients:** except the cilantro, toss, put the pan in the air fryer and cook at 380°F for 15 minutes
Divide between plates and serve with cilantro sprinkled on top.
Nutrition: Calories: 141; Fat: 3g; Fiber: 2g; Carbs: 4g; Protein: 5g

Butter Broccoli

Preparation Time: 20 minutes
Servings: 4
Ingredients:
1 lb. broccoli florets
½ tbsp. butter; melted
1 tsp. sweet paprika
A pinch of salt and black pepper
Directions:
Take a bowl and mix the broccoli with the rest of the **Ingredients:** and toss.
Put the broccoli in your air fryer's basket, cook at 350°F for 15 minutes, divide between plates and serve
Nutrition: Calories: 130; Fat: 3g; Fiber: 3g; Carbs: 4g; Protein: 8g

Garlic Tomatoes

Preparation Time: 20 minutes
Servings: 4
Ingredients:
1 lb. cherry tomatoes; halved
6 garlic cloves; minced
1 tbsp. olive oil
1 tbsp. dill; chopped.
1 tbsp. balsamic vinegar
Salt and black pepper to taste.
Directions:
In a pan that fits the air fryer, combine all the **Ingredients:**, toss gently.
Put the pan in the air fryer and cook at 380°F for 15 minutes
Divide between plates and serve.
Nutrition: Calories: 121; Fat: 3g; Fiber: 2g; Carbs: 4g; Protein: 6g

Spicy Olives and Avocado

Preparation Time: 20 minutes
Servings: 4
Ingredients:
2 small avocados, pitted; peeled and sliced
¼ cup cherry tomatoes; halved
2 cups kalamata olives, pitted
1 tbsp. coconut oil; melted
Juice of 1 lime
Directions:
In a pan that fits the air fryer, combine the olives with the other **Ingredients:**, toss.
Put the pan in your air fryer and cook at 370°F for 15 minutes
Divide the mix between plates and serve.
Nutrition: Calories: 153; Fat: 3g; Fiber: 3g; Carbs: 4g; Protein: 6g

Kale and Brussels Sprouts

Preparation Time: 20 minutes
Servings: 8
Ingredients:
1 lb. Brussels sprouts, trimmed
3 oz. mozzarella, shredded
2 cups kale, torn
1 tbsp. olive oil
Salt and black pepper to taste.
Directions:
In a pan that fits the air fryer, combine all the **Ingredients:** except the mozzarella and toss.
Put the pan in the air fryer and cook at 380°F for 15 minutes
Divide between plates, sprinkle the cheese on top and serve.
Nutrition: Calories: 170; Fat: 5g; Fiber: 3g; Carbs: 4g; Protein: 7g

Balsamic Kale

Preparation Time: 14 minutes
Servings: 6
Ingredients:
2 ½ lb. kale leaves
3 garlic cloves; minced
2 tbsp. olive oil
2 tbsp. balsamic vinegar
Salt and black pepper to taste.
Directions:
In a pan that fits the air fryer, combine all the **Ingredients:** and toss.
Put the pan in your air fryer and cook at 300°F for 12 minutes. Divide between plates and serve
Nutrition: Calories: 122; Fat: 4g; Fiber: 3g; Carbs: 4g; Protein: 5g

Kale and Bell Peppers

Preparation Time: 15 minutes
Servings: 4
Ingredients:
1 ½ cups avocado, peeled, pitted and cubed
2 cups kale, torn
¼ cup olive oil

1 cup red bell pepper; sliced
1 tbsp. white vinegar
2 tbsp. lime juice
1 tbsp. mustard
A pinch of salt and black pepper

Directions:

In a pan that fits the air fryer, combine the kale with salt, pepper, avocado and half of the oil, toss.

Put in your air fryer and cook at 360°F for 10 minutes

In a bowl, combine the kale mix with the rest of the **Ingredients:**, toss and serve.

Nutrition: Calories: 131; Fat: 3g; Fiber: 2g; Carbs: 4g; Protein: 5g

Asparagus and Yogurt Sauce

Preparation Time: 14 minutes
Servings: 4
Ingredients:

1 lb. asparagus, trimmed
2 garlic cloves; minced
¼ cup chives; chopped
¼ cup lemon juice
1 cup Greek yogurt
1 cup basil; chopped
½ cup parsley; chopped
2 tbsp. olive oil
1 tsp. garlic powder
1 tsp. oregano; dried
A pinch of salt and black pepper

Directions:

Take a bowl and mix the asparagus with the oil, salt, pepper, oregano and garlic powder and toss.

Put the asparagus in the air fryer's basket and cook at 400°F for 10 minutes

Meanwhile, in a blender, mix the yogurt with basil, chives, parsley, lemon juice and garlic cloves and pulse well

Divide the asparagus between plates, drizzle the sauce all over and serve.

Nutrition: Calories: 194; Fat: 6g; Fiber: 2g; Carbs: 4g; Protein: 8g

Italian Asparagus

Preparation Time: 15 minutes
Servings: 4
Ingredients:

1 lb. asparagus, trimmed
2 cups cherry tomatoes; halved
2 cups mozzarella, shredded
½ cup balsamic vinegar
2 tbsp. olive oil
A pinch of salt and black pepper

Directions:

In a pan that fits your air fryer, mix the asparagus with the rest of the **Ingredients:** except the mozzarella and toss

Put the pan in the air fryer and cook at 400°F for 10 minutes. Divide between plates and serve

Nutrition: Calories: 200; Fat: 6g; Fiber: 2g; Carbs: 3g; Protein: 6g

Tomato, Avocado and Green Beans

Preparation Time: 20 minutes
Servings: 4
Ingredients:
¼ lb. green beans, trimmed and halved
1 avocado, peeled, pitted and cubed
1 pint mixed cherry tomatoes; halved
2 tbsp. olive oil
Directions:
In a pan that fits your air fryer, mix the tomatoes with the rest of the **Ingredients:**, toss.
Put the pan in the machine and cook at 360°F for 15 minutes. Transfer to bowls and serve
Nutrition: Calories: 151; Fat: 3g; Fiber: 2g; Carbs: 4g; Protein: 4g

Kale and Olives

Preparation Time: 20 minutes
Servings: 4
Ingredients:
1 an ½ lb. kale, torn
1 tbsp. hot paprika
2 tbsp. olive oil
2 tbsp. black olives, pitted and sliced
Salt and black pepper to taste.
Directions:
In a pan that fits the air fryer, combine all the **Ingredients:** and toss.
Put the pan in your air fryer, cook at 370°F for 15 minutes, divide between plates and serve
Nutrition: Calories: 154; Fat: 3g; Fiber: 2g; Carbs: 4g; Protein: 6g

Lemon Endives

Preparation Time: 20 minutes
Servings: 4
Ingredients:
12 endives, trimmed
3 tbsp. ghee; melted
1 tbsp. lemon juice
A pinch of salt and black pepper
Directions:
Take a bowl and mix the endives with the ghee, salt, pepper and lemon juice and toss.
Put the endives in the fryer's basket and cook at 350°F for 15 minutes
Divide between plates and serve.
Nutrition: Calories: 163; Fat: 4g; Fiber: 3g; Carbs: 5g; Protein: 6g

Italian Asparagus Mix

Preparation Time: 5 minutes
Cooking time: 10 minutes
Servings: 4
Ingredients:
1 pound asparagus, trimmed
2 tablespoons olive oil
A pinch of salt and black pepper
2 cups mozzarella, shredded
½ cup balsamic vinegar

2 cups cherry tomatoes, halved

Directions:

In a pan that fits your air fryer, mix the asparagus with the rest of the **Ingredients:** except the mozzarella and toss.

Put the pan in the air fryer and cook at 400 degrees F for 10 minutes.

Divide between plates and serve.

Nutrition: calories 200, fat 6, fiber 2, carbs 3, protein 6

Roasted Asparagus

Preparation Time: 5 minutes
Cooking time: 10 minutes
Servings: 4
Ingredients:

1 pound asparagus, trimmed
3 tablespoons olive oil
A pinch of salt and black pepper
1 tablespoon sweet paprika

Directions:

In a bowl, mix the asparagus with the rest of the **Ingredients:** and toss.

Put the asparagus in your air fryer's basket and cook at 400 degrees F for 10 minutes.

Divide between plates and serve.

Nutrition: calories 200, fat 5, fiber 2, carbs 4, protein 6

Asparagus and Yogurt Sauce

Preparation Time: 4 minutes
Cooking time: 10 minutes
Servings: 4
Ingredients:

1 pound asparagus, trimmed
2 tablespoons olive oil
A pinch of salt and black pepper
1 teaspoon garlic powder
1 teaspoon oregano, dried
1 cup Greek yogurt
1 cup basil, chopped
½ cup parsley, chopped
¼ cup chives, chopped
¼ cup lemon juice
2 garlic cloves, minced

Directions:

In a bowl, mix the asparagus with the oil, salt, pepper, oregano and garlic powder, and toss.

Put the asparagus in the air fryer's basket and cook at 400 degrees F for 10 minutes.

Meanwhile, in a blender, mix the yogurt with basil, chives, parsley, lemon juice and garlic cloves and pulse well.

Divide the asparagus between plates, drizzle the sauce all over and serve.

Nutrition: calories 194, fat 6, fiber 2, carbs 4, protein 8

Asparagus and Tomatoes

Preparation Time: 5 minutes
Cooking time: 10 minutes
Servings: 4
Ingredients:
1 pound asparagus, trimmed
2 cups cherry tomatoes, halved
¼ cup parmesan, grated
½ cup balsamic vinegar
2 tablespoons olive oil
A pinch of salt and black pepper
Directions:
In a bowl, mix the asparagus with the rest of the **Ingredients:** except the parmesan, and toss.
Put the asparagus and tomatoes in your air fryer's basket and cook at 400 degrees F for 10 minutes
Divide between plates and serve with the parmesan sprinkled on top.
Nutrition: calories 173, fat 4, fiber 2, carbs 4, protein 8

Bacon Asparagus Mix

Preparation Time: 5 minutes
Cooking time: 10 minutes
Servings: 4
Ingredients:
2 pounds asparagus, trimmed
2 tablespoons olive oil
1 cup cheddar cheese, shredded
4 garlic cloves, minced
4 bacon slices, cooked and crumbled
Directions:
In a bowl, mix the asparagus with the other **Ingredients:** except the bacon, toss and put in your air fryer's basket.
Cook at 400 degrees F for 10 minutes, divide between plates, sprinkle the bacon on top and serve.
Nutrition: calories 172, fat 6, fiber 2, carbs 5, protein 8

Mustard Asparagus Mix

Preparation Time: 5 minutes
Cooking time: 12 minutes
Servings: 4
Ingredients:
1 pound asparagus, trimmed
2 tablespoons olive oil
¼ cup mustard
3 garlic cloves, minced
½ cup parmesan, grated
Directions:
In a bowl, mix the asparagus with the oil, garlic and mustard and toss really well.
Put the asparagus spears in your air fryer's basket and cook at 400 degrees F for 12 minutes.
Divide between plates, sprinkle the parmesan on top and serve.
Nutrition: calories 162, fat 4, fiber 4, carbs 6, protein 9

Lemon Asparagus

Preparation Time: 5 minutes
Cooking time: 12 minutes
Servings: 4
Ingredients:
1 pound asparagus, trimmed
A pinch of salt and black pepper
2 tablespoons olive oil
3 garlic cloves, minced
3 tablespoons parmesan, grated
Juice of 1 lemon
Directions:
In a bowl, mix the asparagus with the rest of the **Ingredients:** and toss.
Put the asparagus in your air fryer's basket and cook at 390 degrees F for 12 minutes.
Divide between plates and serve.
Nutrition: calories 175, fat 5, fiber 2, carbs 4, protein 8

Broccoli Casserole

Preparation Time: 5 minutes
Cooking time: 30 minutes
Servings: 4
Ingredients:
3 tablespoons ghee, melted
15 ounces coconut cream
2 eggs, whisked
2 cups cheddar, grated
1 cup parmesan, grated
1 tablespoon mustard
1 pound broccoli florets
A pinch of salt and black pepper
1 tablespoon parsley, chopped
Directions:
Grease a baking pan that fits the air fryer with the ghee and arrange the broccoli on the bottom.
Add the cream, mustard, salt, pepper and the eggs and toss.
Sprinkle the cheese on top, put the pan in the air fryer and cook at 380 degrees F for 30 minutes.
Divide between plates and serve.
Nutrition: calories 244, fat 12, fiber 3, carbs 5, protein 12

Vinegar Broccoli Mix

Preparation Time: 5 minutes
Cooking time: 25 minutes
Servings: 4
Ingredients:
1 broccoli head, florets separated
2 shallots, chopped
A pinch of salt and black pepper
½ cup cranberries
½ cup almonds, chopped
6 bacon slices, cooked and crumbled
3 tablespoons balsamic vinegar

Directions:
In a pan that fits the air fryer, combine the broccoli with the rest of the **Ingredients:** and toss.
Put the pan in the air fryer and cook at 380 degrees F for 25 minutes.
Divide between plates and serve.
Nutrition: calories 173, fat 7, fiber 2, carbs 4, protein 8

Broccoli And Tomato Sauce

Preparation Time: 5 minutes
Cooking time: 15 minutes
Servings: 4
Ingredients:
1 broccoli head, florets separated
Salt and black pepper to the taste
½ cup tomato sauce
1 tablespoon sweet paprika
¼ cup scallions, chopped
1 tablespoon olive oil
Directions:
In a pan that fits the air fryer, combine the broccoli with the rest of the **Ingredients:**, toss, put the pan in the fryer and cook at 380 degrees F for 15 minutes.
Divide between plates and serve.
Nutrition: calories 163, fat 5, fiber 2, carbs 4, protein 8

SIDE DISHES AND SNACK

Zucchini Sauté

Preparation Time: 10 minutes
Cooking time: 20 minutes
Servings: 4
Ingredients:
1 pound zucchinis, roughly cubed
1 teaspoon sweet paprika
½ cup heavy cream
3 garlic cloves, minced
1 tablespoon olive oil
Salt and black pepper to the taste
2 tablespoons dill, chopped
Directions:
In your air fryer, combine the zucchinis with the paprika and the other **Ingredients:**, toss gently and cook at 370 degrees F for 20 minutes.
Divide between plates and serve as a side dish.
Nutrition: calories 109, fat 4, fiber 7, carbs 1, protein 2

Cumin Eggplant Mix

Preparation Time: 10 minutes
Cooking time: 20 minutes
Servings: 4
Ingredients:
1 pound eggplant, roughly cubed
1 cup cherry tomatoes, halved
1 red onion, chopped
Salt and black pepper to the taste
2 tablespoons olive oil
½ teaspoon chili powder
½ teaspoon cumin, ground
1 tablespoon chives, chopped
Directions:
Heat up the air fryer with the oil at 350 degrees F, add the eggplants and the other **Ingredients:**, toss gently, and cook for 20 minutes.
Divide the mix between plates and serve as a side dish.
Nutrition: calories 110, fat 5, fiber 3, carbs 13, protein 9

Garlic Kale

Preparation Time: 10 minutes
Cooking time: 20 minutes
Servings: 4
Ingredients:
1 pound kale leaves, torn
1 tablespoon avocado oil
1 teaspoon coriander, ground
1 teaspoon basil, dried
1 tablespoon balsamic vinegar
4 garlic cloves, minced

Salt and black pepper to the taste
Directions:
In your air fryer, combine the kale with the oil and the other **Ingredients:**, toss well and cook them at 370 degrees F for 20 minutes.
Divide the mix between plates and serve as a side dish.
Nutrition: calories 66, fat 5, fiber 8, carbs 11, protein 6

Green Beans Sauté

Preparation Time: 10 minutes
Cooking time: 20 minutes
Servings: 4
Ingredients:
2 pounds green beans, trimmed and halved
Salt and black pepper to the taste
1 tablespoon balsamic vinegar
1 tablespoon dill, chopped
2 tablespoons olive oil
Directions:
In your air fryer's basket, combine the green beans with the vinegar and the other **Ingredients:**, toss and cook at 350 degrees F for 20 minutes.
Divide between plates and serve as a side dish.
Nutrition: calories 133, fat 3, fiber 8, carbs 16, protein 3

Herbed Tomatoes

Preparation Time: 10 minutes
Cooking time: 20 minutes
Servings: 4
Ingredients:
1 pound tomatoes, cut into wedges
2 tablespoons chives, chopped
1 tablespoon oregano, chopped
1 tablespoon balsamic vinegar
1 teaspoon Italian seasoning
A pinch of salt and black pepper
2 tablespoons olive oil
Directions:
In your air fryer's basket, combine the tomatoes with the chives, vinegar and the other **Ingredients:**, toss and cook at 360 degrees F for 20 minutes.
Divide everything between plates and serve as a side dish.
Nutrition: calories 89, fat 7, fiber 9, carbs 4, protein 2

Coriander Potatoes

Preparation Time: 10 minutes
Cooking time: 25 minutes
Servings: 4
Ingredients:
1 pound gold potatoes, peeled and cut into wedges
Salt and black pepper to the taste
1 tablespoon tomato sauce
2 tablespoons coriander, chopped
½ teaspoon garlic powder

1 teaspoon chili powder
1 tablespoon olive oil
Directions:
In a bowl, combine the potatoes with the tomato sauce and the other **Ingredients:**, toss, and transfer to the air fryer's basket.
Cook at 370 degrees F for 25 minutes, divide between plates and serve as a side dish.
Nutrition: calories 210, fat 5, fiber 7, carbs 12, protein 5

Creamy Green Beans and Tomatoes

Preparation Time: 10 minutes
Cooking time: 20 minutes
Servings: 4
Ingredients:
1 pound green beans, trimmed and halved
½ pound cherry tomatoes, halved
2 tablespoons olive oil
1 teaspoon oregano, dried
1 teaspoon basil, dried
Salt and black pepper to the taste
1 cup heavy cream
½ tablespoon cilantro, chopped
Directions:
In your air fryer's pan, combine the green beans with the tomatoes and the other **Ingredients:**, toss and cook at 360 degrees F for 20 minutes.
Divide the mix between plates and serve.
Nutrition: calories 174, fat 5, fiber 7, carbs 11, protein 4

Buttery Artichokes

Preparation Time: 10 minutes
Cooking time: 20 minutes
Servings: 4
Ingredients:
4 artichokes, trimmed and halved
3 garlic cloves, minced
1 tablespoon olive oil
Salt and black pepper to the taste
4 tablespoons butter, melted
¼ teaspoon cumin, ground
1 tablespoon lemon zest, grated
Directions:
In a bowl, combine the artichokes with the oil, garlic and the other **Ingredients:**, toss well and transfer them to the air fryer's basket.
Cook for 20 minutes at 370 degrees F, divide between plates and serve as a side dish.
Nutrition: calories 214, fat 5, fiber 8, carbs 12, protein 5

Sweet Potato and Eggplant Mix

Preparation Time: 10 minutes
Cooking time: 20 minutes
Servings: 4
Ingredients:
2 sweet potatoes, peeled and cut into medium wedges

2 eggplants, roughly cubed
1 tablespoon avocado oil
Juice of 1 lemon
4 garlic cloves, minced
1 teaspoon nutmeg, ground
Salt and black pepper to the taste
1 tablespoon rosemary, chopped

Directions:

In your air fryer, combine the potatoes with the eggplants and the other **Ingredients:**, toss and cook at 370 degrees F for 20 minutes.

Divide the mix between plates and serve as a side dish.

Nutrition: calories 182, fat 6, fiber 3, carbs 11, protein 5

Peppers and Tomatoes Mix

Preparation Time: 5 minutes
Cooking time: 20 minutes
Servings: 4

Ingredients:

1 tablespoon olive oil
1 red onion, sliced
1 pound cherry tomatoes, halved
1 red bell pepper, cut into medium strips
1 green bell pepper, cut in medium strips
1 teaspoon chili powder
1 teaspoon garam masala
Salt and black pepper to the taste

Directions:

In your air fryer, combine the tomatoes with the bell peppers and the other **Ingredients:**, toss and cook at 370 degrees F for 20 minutes.

Divide the mix between plates and serve as a side dish.

Nutrition: calories 172, fat 5, fiber 4, carbs 7, protein 4

Chives Carrots and Onions

Preparation Time: 5 minutes
Cooking time: 20 minutes
Servings: 4

Ingredients:

1 pound baby carrots, peeled
2 red onions, sliced
1 tablespoon lime zest, grated
1 tablespoon balsamic vinegar
2 tablespoons chives, chopped

Directions:

In your air fryer's basket, combine the carrots with the onions and the other **Ingredients:**, toss and cook at 320 degrees F for 20 minutes.

Divide between plates and serve as a side dish.

Nutrition: calories 132, fat 4, fiber 3, carbs 11, protein 4

Cilantro Brussels Sprouts

Preparation Time: 5 minutes
Cooking time: 25 minutes
Servings: 4
Ingredients:
2 pounds Brussels sprouts, trimmed and halved
1 tablespoon olive oil
2 tablespoons maple syrup
1 tablespoon cilantro, chopped
1 tablespoon sweet paprika
A pinch of salt and black pepper
Directions:
In your air fryer's basket, combine the sprouts with the oil, maple syrup and the remaining **Ingredients:**, toss and cook at 360 degrees F for 25 minutes.
Divide between plates and serve as a side dish.
Nutrition: calories 174, fat 5, fiber 3, carbs 11, protein 4

Garlic Beets

Preparation Time: 10 minutes
Cooking time: 25 minutes
Servings: 4
Ingredients:
2 pounds beets, peeled and roughly cubed
A pinch of salt and black pepper
1 teaspoon chili powder
4 garlic cloves, minced
1 tablespoon olive oil
Directions:
In your air fryer's basket, combine the beets with salt, pepper and the other **Ingredients:**, toss and cook at 370 degrees F for 25 minutes.
Divide the beets between plates and serve as a side dish.
Nutrition: calories 171, fat 4, fiber 2, carbs 13, protein 3

Ginger Mushrooms

Preparation Time: 10 minutes
Cooking time: 20 minutes
Servings: 4
Ingredients:
2 tablespoons olive oil
2 tablespoons balsamic vinegar
2 pounds white mushrooms, halved
1 tablespoon ginger, grated
A pinch of salt and black pepper
1 teaspoon cumin, ground
Directions:
In your air fryer's basket, combine the mushrooms with the oil, vinegar and the other **Ingredients:**, toss and cook at 360 degrees F for 20 minutes.
Divide the mix between plates and serve.
Nutrition: calories 182, fat 3, fiber 2, carbs 8, protein 4

Masala Potatoes

Preparation Time: 10 minutes
Cooking time: 20 minutes
Servings: 4
Ingredients:
2 pounds gold potatoes, peeled and roughly cubed
1 tablespoon olive oil
1 teaspoon garlic powder
1 teaspoon garam masala
Juice of 1 lime
A pinch of salt and black pepper
Directions:
In your air fryer's basket, combine the potatoes with the garam masala and the other **Ingredients:**, toss and cook at 370 degrees F for 20 minutes.
Divide the mix between plates and serve.
Nutrition: calories 182, fat 4, fiber 7, carbs 12, protein 4

Lime Broccoli

Preparation Time: 10 minutes
Cooking time: 20 minutes
Servings: 4
Ingredients:
1 tablespoon avocado oil
1 pound broccoli florets
1 tablespoon ginger, grated
A pinch of salt and black pepper
Juice of 1 lime
Directions:
In your air fryer's basket, combine the broccoli with the oil and the other **Ingredients:**, toss and cook at 370 degrees F for 20 minutes.
Divide the mix between plates and serve.
Nutrition: calories 182, fat 4, fiber 3, carbs 11, protein 4

Rosemary Mustard Beets

Preparation Time: 10 minutes
Cooking time: 30 minutes
Servings: 4
Ingredients:
1 pound beets, peeled and roughly cubed
1 tablespoon mustard
1 tablespoon rosemary, chopped
Salt and black pepper the taste
2 garlic cloves, minced
Directions:
In your air fryer's basket, combine the beets with the mustard and the other **Ingredients:**, toss and cook at 370 degrees F for 30 minutes.
Divide between plates and serve as a side dish.
Nutrition: calories 190, fat 4, fiber 4, carbs 14, protein 4

Thyme Parsnips Mix

Preparation Time: 10 minutes
Cooking time: 15 minutes
Servings: 4
Ingredients:
4 parsnips, cut into medium sticks
Salt and black pepper to the taste
2 tablespoons thyme, chopped
2 tablespoons olive oil
1 teaspoon sweet paprika
½ cup tomato sauce
Directions:
In your air fryer's pan, combine the parsnips with salt, pepper and the other **Ingredients:**, toss and cook at 350 degrees F for 15 minutes.
Divide between plates and serve as a side dish.
Nutrition: calories 160, fat 3, fiber 4, carbs 7, protein 3

Sprouts and Mushrooms Mix

Preparation Time: 5 minutes
Cooking time: 20 minutes
Servings: 4
Ingredients:
1 cup white mushrooms, halved
1 pound Brussels sprouts, trimmed and halved
1 red onion, sliced
2 tablespoons olive oil
Salt and black pepper to the taste
½ teaspoon rosemary, dried
2 tablespoons cilantro, chopped
Directions:
In your air fryer's basket, combine the white mushrooms with the sprouts and the other **Ingredients:**, toss and cook at 380 degrees F for 20 minutes.
Divide the mix between plates and serve as a side dish.
Nutrition: calories 202, fat 6, fiber 1, carbs 16, protein 4

Tomato and Squash Mix

Preparation Time: 10 minutes
Cooking time: 20 minutes
Servings: 4
Ingredients:
2 tablespoons olive oil
½ pound cherry tomatoes, halved
1 butternut squash, peeled and roughly cubed
1 teaspoon turmeric powder
1 teaspoon chili powder
Salt and black pepper to the taste
1 tablespoon cilantro, chopped
Directions:
Heat up the air fryer with the oil at 360 degrees F, add the tomatoes, squash and the other **Ingredients:**, toss and cook for 20 minutes.

Divide everything between plates and serve as a side dish.
Nutrition: calories 200, fat 4, fiber 1, carbs 15, protein 4

Parsley Mushrooms

Preparation Time: 10 minutes
Cooking time: 15 minutes
Servings: 4
Ingredients:
1 pound baby Bella mushroom caps
1 teaspoon cumin, ground
1 tablespoon olive oil
2 teaspoons chili flakes, crushed
1 tablespoon parsley, chopped
Salt and black pepper to the taste
Directions:
In your air fryer's basket, combine the mushroom caps with the cumin and the other **Ingredients:**, toss and cook at 380 degrees F for 15 minutes.
Divide between plates and serve as a side dish.
Nutrition: calories 161, fat 7, fiber 1, carbs 12, protein 6

Paprika Corn and Kale

Preparation Time: 10 minutes
Cooking time: 15 minutes
Servings: 4
Ingredients:
2 cups fresh corn
1 cup baby kale
Salt and black pepper to the taste
2 teaspoons olive oil
Juice of 1 lime
1 teaspoon turmeric powder
2 teaspoon smoked paprika
Directions:
In your air fryer, combine the corn with the kale, oil and the other **Ingredients:**, toss and cook at 360 degrees F for 15 minutes.
Divide between plates and serve.
Nutrition: calories 180, fat 7, fiber 2, carbs 12, protein 6

Garlic Kale Mix

Preparation Time: 10 minutes
Cooking time: 15 minutes
Servings: 4
Ingredients:
1 pound kale leaves, torn
1 teaspoon rosemary, dried
1 teaspoon fenugreek seeds, crushed
Salt and black pepper to the taste
2 tablespoons olive oil
1 tablespoon garlic, minced

Directions:
In your air fryer, combine the kale with the rosemary, garlic and the other **Ingredients:**, toss and cook at 360 degrees F for 15 minutes.
Divide the mix between plates and serve as a side dish.
Nutrition: calories 173, fat 3, fiber 2, carbs 16, protein 4

Red Cabbage and Sprouts

Preparation Time: 10 minutes
Cooking time: 20 minute
Servings: 4
Ingredients:
1 red cabbage head, shredded
½ pound Brussels sprouts, trimmed and halved
1 red onion, chopped
2 tablespoons olive oil
1 teaspoon sweet paprika
Salt and black pepper to the taste
4 bacon slices, cooked and crumbled
1 tablespoon chives, chopped
Directions:
Heat up the air fryer with the oil at 360 degrees F, add the onion, cabbage and the other **Ingredients:**, toss and cook for 20 minutes.
Divide between plates and serve as a side dish.
Nutrition: calories 208, fat 10, fiber 4, carbs 12, protein 4

Walnuts Rice Mix

Preparation Time: 10 minutes
Cooking time: 25 minutes
Servings: 4
Ingredients:
1 red onion, chopped
2 cups wild rice
4 cups chicken stock
1 teaspoon olive oil
1 teaspoon garlic, minced
1 teaspoon olive oil
Salt and black pepper to the taste
1 tablespoon parsley, chopped
½ cup walnuts, chopped
Directions:
In your air fryer's pan, combine the rice with the stock, onion and the other **Ingredients:**, toss and cook at 380 degrees F for 25 minutes.
Divide between plates and serve as a side dish.
Nutrition: calories 200, fat 4, fiber 6, carbs 16, protein 4

Cranberry Barley Mix

Preparation Time: 10 minutes
Cooking time: 25 minutes
Servings: 4
Ingredients:
2 cups barley

3 cups chicken stock
½ cup cranberries
2 garlic cloves, minced
1 tablespoon olive oil
Salt and black pepper to the taste
1 teaspoon turmeric powder
1 teaspoon chili powder
1 tablespoon parsley, chopped

Directions:

In your air fryer's pan, combine the barley with the stock, cranberries and the other **Ingredients:**, toss and cook at 370 degrees F for 25 minutes.

Divide the mix between plates and serve as a side dish.

Nutrition: calories 171, fat 4, fiber 8, carbs 16, protein 7

Rice and Mushrooms Mix

Preparation Time: 10 minutes
Cooking time: 20 minutes
Servings: 4

Ingredients:

2 cups white rice
4 cups chicken stock, heated up
1 red onion, chopped
1 tablespoon avocado oil
1 cup white mushrooms, sliced
2 tablespoons parmesan, grated
1 tablespoon chives, chopped

Directions:

In your air fryer's pan, combine the rice with the stock and the other **Ingredients:**, stir, and cook at 360 degrees F for 20 minutes.

Divide between plates and serve.

Nutrition: calories 261, fat 5, fiber 8, carbs 15, protein 5

Pumpkin and Zucchini Mix

Preparation Time: 5 minutes
Cooking time: 20 minutes
Servings: 4

Ingredients:

1 tablespoon olive oil
3 scallions, chopped
2 garlic cloves, minced
2 zucchinis, cubed
1 cup pumpkin, peeled and cubed
½ teaspoon nutmeg, ground
½ teaspoon ginger, grated
A pinch of salt and black pepper
1 tablespoon chives, chopped

Directions:

Heat up the air fryer with the oil at 360 degrees F, add the garlic, scallions, zucchinis and the other **Ingredients:**, toss and cook for 20 minutes.

Divide between plates and serve as a side dish.

Nutrition: calories 251, fat 6, fiber 8, carbs 16, protein 6

Sage Potatoes

Preparation Time: 5 minutes
Cooking time: 20 minutes
Servings: 4
Ingredients:
1 tablespoon olive oil
2 pounds red potatoes, peeled and cut into wedges
Salt and black pepper to the taste
1 teaspoon sage, dried
½ cup parmesan, grated
2 tablespoon butter, melted
Directions:
Heat up the air fryer with the oil and the butter at 360 degrees F, add the potatoes and the other **Ingredients:**, toss and cook for 20 minutes.
Divide between plates and serve as a side dish.
Nutrition: calories 251, fat 6, fiber 5, carbs 16, protein 6

Almond Spinach Mix

Preparation Time: 10 minutes
Cooking time: 12 minutes
Servings: 4
Ingredients:
1 tablespoon olive oil
2 spring onions, chopped
1 pound baby spinach
½ cup almonds, chopped
Salt and black pepper to the taste
1 teaspoon cumin, ground
1 tablespoon chives, chopped
Directions:
In your air fryer, combine the spinach with the oil, almonds and the other **Ingredients:**, toss and cook at 360 degrees F for 20 minutes.
Divide between plates and serve as a side dish.
Nutrition: calories 251, fat 4, fiber 3, carbs 13, protein 6

Mint Beets Mix

Preparation Time: 10 minutes
Cooking time: 25 minutes
Servings: 4
Ingredients:
1 tablespoon olive oil
4 beets, peeled and roughly cubed
1 tablespoon lemon juice
1 teaspoon sweet paprika
1 tablespoon mint, chopped
Salt and black pepper to the taste
¼ cup green onions, chopped
Directions:
In your the fryer, combine the beets with the oil, lemon juice and the other **Ingredients:**, toss and cook at 360 degrees F for 25 minutes.

Divide between plates and serve as a side dish.
Nutrition: calories 200, fat 5, fiber 5, carbs 9, protein 5

Cauliflower Rice

Preparation Time: 10 minutes
Cooking time: 20 minutes
Servings: 4
Ingredients:
2 tablespoons olive oil
Salt and black pepper to the taste
2 cups cauliflower florets
1 cup wild rice
2 cups chicken stock
½ cup parmesan, grated
2 garlic cloves, minced
2 tablespoons parsley, chopped
Directions:
In your air fryer's pan, combine the rice with the stock and the other **Ingredients:**, toss and cook at 370 degrees F for 20 minutes.
Divide between plates and serve as a side dish.
Nutrition: calories 200, fat 6, fiber 5, carbs 15, protein 5

Creamy Endives

Preparation Time: 10 minutes
Cooking time: 20 minutes
Servings: 4
Ingredients:
1 tablespoon olive oil
4 endives, shredded
2 garlic cloves, minced
¼ cup chicken stock
¼ cup heavy cream
1 tablespoon parmesan, grated
Salt and black pepper to the taste
1 tablespoon chives, chopped
Directions:
In your air fryer's pan, combine the endives with the garlic and the other **Ingredients:**, toss and cook at 360 degrees F for 20 minutes.
Divide between plates and serve as a side dish.
Nutrition: calories 215, fat 4, fiber 6, carbs 14, protein 4

Chicken Party Meatballs

Preparation Time: 25 minutes
Servings: 12
Ingredients:
2 lb. chicken breast, skinless; boneless and ground
2 garlic cloves; minced
2 spring onions; chopped.
¾ cup almond meal
6 tbsp. hot sauce
2 tbsp. ghee; melted

Cooking spray
A pinch of salt and black pepper
Directions:
Take a bowl and mix all the **Ingredients:** except the cooking spray, stir well and shape medium meatballs out of this mix
Arrange the meatballs in your air fryer's basket, grease them with cooking spray and cook at 360°F for 20 minutes.
Nutrition: Calories: 257; Fat: 14g; Fiber: 1g; Carbs: 3g; Protein: 17g

Smoked Salmon Bites

Preparation Time: 15 minutes
Servings: 12
Ingredients:
4 oz. smoked salmon, skinless; boneless and chopped.
2 avocados, peeled, pitted and mashed
2 tbsp. coconut cream
1 tsp. dill; chopped.
1 tsp. avocado oil
A pinch of salt and black pepper
Directions:
Take a bowl and mix all the **Ingredients:**, stir well and shape medium balls out of this mix.
Place them in your air fryer's basket and cook at 350°F for 10 minutes
Nutrition: Calories: 100; Fat: 2g; Fiber: 1g; Carbs: 2g; Protein: 2g

Shrimp and Mushrooms Dip

Preparation Time: 25 minutes
Servings: 4
Ingredients:
1 lb. shrimp, peeled, deveined and minced
¼ lb. mushrooms; minced
½ cup mozzarella; shredded
4 garlic cloves; minced
1 tbsp. parsley; chopped.
2 tbsp. ghee; melted
Salt and black pepper to taste.
Directions:
Take a bowl and mix all the **Ingredients:**, stir well, divide into small ramekins and place them in your air fryer's basket
Cook at 360°F for 20 minutes and serve as a party dip.
Nutrition: Calories: 271; Fat: 15g; Fiber: 3g; Carbs: 4g; Protein: 14g

Avocado Balls

Preparation Time: 10 minutes
Servings: 4
Ingredients:
1 avocado, peeled, pitted and mashed
4 bacon slices, cooked and crumbled
2 spring onions; minced
1 chili pepper; chopped.
¼ cup ghee; melted
2 garlic cloves; minced

2 tbsp. cilantro
1 tbsp. lime juice
A pinch of salt and black pepper
Cooking spray

Directions:

Take a bowl and mix all the **Ingredients:** except the cooking spray, stir well and shape medium balls out of this mix

Place them in your air fryer's basket, grease with cooking spray and cook at 370°F for 5 minutes.

Nutrition: Calories: 160; Fat: 6g; Fiber: 3g; Carbs: 4g; Protein: 6g

Pork Rind Nachos

Preparation Time: 10 minutes
Servings: 2
Ingredients:

1 oz. pork rinds.
4 oz. shredded cooked chicken.
¼ cup guacamole.
½ cup shredded Monterey jack cheese.
¼ cup full-fat sour cream.
¼ cup sliced pickled jalapeños.

Directions:

Place pork rinds into 6-inch round baking pan. Cover with shredded chicken and Monterey jack cheese. Place pan into the air fryer basket.

Adjust the temperature to 370 Degrees F and set the timer for 5 minutes or until cheese is melted. Top with jalapeños, guacamole and sour cream. Serve immediately.

Nutrition: Calories: 395; Protein: 31g; Fiber: 2g; Fat: 25g; Carbs: 0g

Cilantro Dip

Preparation Time: 13 minutes
Servings: 6
Ingredients:

½ cup cashews, soaked in water for 4 hours and drained
2 garlic cloves; minced
2 tbsp. coconut milk
3 tbsp. cilantro; chopped.
1 tsp. lime juice
A pinch of salt and black pepper

Directions:

In a blender, combine all the **Ingredients:**, pulse well and transfer to a ramekin.

Put the ramekin in your air fryer's basket and cook at 350°F for 8 minutes. Serve as a dip

Nutrition: Calories: 144; Fat: 2g; Fiber: 1g; Carbs: 3g; Protein: 4g

Radish Chips

Preparation Time: 20 minutes
Servings: 4
Ingredients:

16 oz. radishes, thinly sliced
2 tbsp. coconut oil; melted
A pinch of salt and black pepper

Directions:
Take a bowl and mix the radish slices with salt, pepper and the oil, toss well, place them in your air fryer's basket and cook at 400°F for 15 minutes, flipping them halfway
Nutrition: Calories: 174; Fat: 5g; Fiber: 1g; Carbs: 3g; Protein: 6g

Chili Meatballs

Preparation Time: 25 minutes
Servings: 12
Ingredients:
1 lb. pork meat, ground
3 spring onions; minced
2 garlic cloves; minced
1 chili pepper; minced
3 tbsp. cilantro; chopped.
1 tbsp. ginger; grated
1 ½ tbsp. coconut aminos
A pinch of salt and black pepper
Cooking spray
Directions:
Take a bowl and mix all the **Ingredients:** except the cooking spray, stir really well and shape medium meatballs out of this mix
Arrange them in your air fryer's basket, grease with cooking spray and cook at 380°F for 20 minutes.
Nutrition: Calories: 200; Fat: 12g; Fiber: 2g; Carbs: 3g; Protein: 14g

Party Pork Skewers

Preparation Time: 30 minutes
Servings: 4
Ingredients:
½ lb. pork shoulder; cubed
¼ cup olive oil
¼ cup green bell peppers; chopped.
2 garlic cloves; minced
1 ½ tbsp. lemon juice
1 tbsp. cilantro; chopped.
1 tbsp. coconut oil; melted
2 tbsp. parsley; chopped.
¼ tsp. sweet paprika
¼ tsp. cumin, ground
A pinch of salt and black pepper
Directions:
In a blender, combine the olive oil with bell peppers, lemon juice, cilantro, parsley, garlic, salt and pepper and pulse well.
Thread the meat onto the skewers, sprinkle cumin and paprika all over and rub with the coconut oil
In a bowl mix the pork skewers with the herbed mix and rub well. Place the skewers in your air fryer's basket, cook at 370°F for 10 minutes on each side and serve as an appetizer.
Nutrition: Calories: 249; Fat: 16g; Fiber: 2g; Carbs: 3g; Protein: 17g

Brussels Sprouts Wraps

Preparation Time: 25 minutes
Servings: 12
Ingredients:
12 Brussels sprouts
12 bacon strips
A drizzle of olive oil
Directions:
Wrap each Brussels sprouts in a bacon strip, brush them with some oil.
Put them in your air fryer's basket and cook at 350°F for 20 minutes
Nutrition: Calories: 140; Fat: 5g; Fiber: 2g; Carbs: 4g; Protein: 4g

Bacon Snack

Preparation Time: 15 minutes
Servings: 4
Ingredients:
1 cup dark chocolate; melted
4 bacon slices; halved
A pinch of pink salt
Directions:
Dip each bacon slice in some chocolate, sprinkle pink salt over them.
Put them in your air fryer's basket and cook at 350°F for 10 minutes
Nutrition: Calories: 151; Fat: 4g; Fiber: 2g; Carbs: 4g; Protein: 8g

Shrimp Snack

Preparation Time: 15 minutes
Servings: 4
Ingredients:
1 lb. shrimp; peeled and deveined
¼ cup olive oil
3 garlic cloves; minced
¼ tsp. cayenne pepper
Juice of ½ lemon
A pinch of salt and black pepper
Directions:
In a pan that fits your air fryer, mix all the **Ingredients:**, toss,
Introduce in the fryer and cook at 370°F for 10 minutes. Serve as a snack
Nutrition: Calories: 242; Fat: 14g; Fiber: 2g; Carbs: 3g; Protein: 17g

Avocado Wraps

Preparation Time: 20 minutes
Servings: 4
Ingredients:
2 avocados, peeled, pitted and cut into 12 wedges
1 tbsp. ghee; melted
12 bacon strips
Directions:
Wrap each avocado wedge in a bacon strip, brush them with the ghee.
Put them in your air fryer's basket and cook at 360°F for 15 minutes. Serve as an appetizer
Nutrition: Calories: 161; Fat: 4g; Fiber: 2g; Carbs: 4g; Protein: 6g

Cheesy Meatballs

Preparation Time: 30 minutes
Servings: 16 meatballs
Ingredients:
1 lb. 80/20 ground beef.
3 oz. low-moisture, whole-milk mozzarella, cubed
1 large egg.
½ cup low-carb, no-sugar-added pasta sauce.
¼ cup grated Parmesan cheese.
¼ cup blanched finely ground almond flour.
¼ tsp. onion powder.
1 tsp. dried parsley.
½ tsp. garlic powder.
Directions:
Take a large bowl, add ground beef, almond flour, parsley, garlic powder, onion powder and egg. Fold **Ingredients:** together until fully combined
Form the mixture into 2-inch balls and use your thumb or a spoon to create an indent in the center of each meatball. Place a cube of cheese in the center and form the ball around it.
Place the meatballs into the air fryer, working in batches if necessary. Adjust the temperature to 350 Degrees F and set the timer for 15 minutes
Meatballs will be slightly crispy on the outside and fully cooked when at least 180 Degrees F internally.
When they are finished cooking, toss the meatballs in the sauce and sprinkle with grated Parmesan for serving.
Nutrition: Calories: 447; Protein: 26g; Fiber: 8g; Fat: 27g; Carbs: 4g

Tuna Appetizer

Preparation Time: 15 minutes
Servings: 2
Ingredients:
1 lb. tuna, skinless; boneless and cubed
3 scallion stalks; minced
1 chili pepper; minced
2 tomatoes; cubed
1 tbsp. coconut aminos
2 tbsp. olive oil
1 tbsp. coconut cream
1 tsp. sesame seeds
Directions:
In a pan that fits your air fryer, mix all the **Ingredients:** except the sesame seeds, toss, introduce in the fryer and cook at 360°F for 10 minutes
Divide into bowls and serve as an appetizer with sesame seeds sprinkled on top.
Nutrition: Calories: 231; Fat: 18g; Fiber: 3g; Carbs: 4g; Protein: 18g

Cheese and Leeks Dip

Preparation Time: 17 minutes
Servings: 6
Ingredients:
2 spring onions; minced
4 leeks; sliced

¼ cup coconut cream
3 tbsp. coconut milk
2 tbsp. butter; melted
Salt and white pepper to the taste
Directions:
In a pan that fits your air fryer, mix all the **Ingredients:** and whisk them well.
Introduce the pan in the fryer and cook at 390°F for 12 minutes. Divide into bowls and serve
Nutrition: Calories: 204; Fat: 12g; Fiber: 2g; Carbs: 4g; Protein: 14g

Cucumber Salsa

Preparation Time: 10 minutes
Servings: 4
Ingredients:
1 ½ lb. cucumbers; sliced
2 red chili peppers; chopped.
2 tomatoes cubed
2 spring onions; chopped.
1 tbsp. balsamic vinegar
2 tbsp. ginger; grated
A drizzle of olive oil
Directions:
In a pan that fits your air fryer, mix all the **Ingredients:**, toss, introduce in the fryer and cook at 340°F for 5 minutes
Divide into bowls and serve cold as an appetizer.
Nutrition: Calories: 150; Fat: 2g; Fiber: 1g; Carbs: 2g; Protein: 4g

Chicken Cubes

Preparation Time: 25 minutes
Servings: 4
Ingredients:
1 lb. chicken breasts, skinless; boneless and cubed
2 eggs
¾ cup coconut flakes
2 tsp. garlic powder
Cooking spray
Salt and black pepper to taste.
Directions:
Put the coconut in a bowl and mix the eggs with garlic powder, salt and pepper in a second one.
Dredge the chicken cubes in eggs and then in coconut and arrange them all in your air fryer's basket
Grease with cooking spray, cook at 370°F for 20 minutes. Arrange the chicken bites on a platter and serve as an appetizer.
Nutrition: Calories: 202; Fat: 12g; Fiber: 2g; Carbs: 4g; Protein: 7g

Salmon Spread

Preparation Time: 11 minutes
Servings: 4
Ingredients:
8 oz. cream cheese, soft
½ cup coconut cream
4 oz. smoked salmon, skinless; boneless and minced

2 tbsp. lemon juice
1 tbsp. chives; chopped.
A pinch of salt and black pepper
Directions:
Take a bowl and mix all the **Ingredients:** and whisk them really well.
Transfer the mix to a ramekin, place it in your air fryer's basket and cook at 360°F for 6 minutes
Nutrition: Calories: 180; Fat: 7g; Fiber: 1g; Carbs: 5g; Protein: 7g

Crustless Pizza

Preparation Time: 10 minutes
Servings: 1
Ingredients:
2 slices sugar-free bacon; cooked and crumbled
7 slices pepperoni
½ cup shredded mozzarella cheese
¼ cup cooked ground sausage
2 tbsp. low-carb, sugar-free pizza sauce, for dipping
1 tbsp. grated Parmesan cheese
Directions:
Cover the bottom of a 6-inch cake pan with mozzarella. Place pepperoni, sausage and bacon on top of cheese and sprinkle with Parmesan
Place pan into the air fryer basket. Adjust the temperature to 400 Degrees F and set the timer for 5 minutes.
Remove when cheese is bubbling and golden. Serve warm with pizza sauce for dipping.
Nutrition: Calories: 466; Protein: 21g; Fiber: 5g; Fat: 30g; Carbs: 2g

Olives and Zucchini Cakes

Preparation Time: 17 minutes
Servings: 6
Ingredients:
3 spring onions; chopped.
½ cup kalamata olives, pitted and minced
3 zucchinis; grated
½ cup parsley; chopped.
½ cup almond flour
1 egg
Cooking spray
Salt and black pepper to taste.
Directions:
Take a bowl and mix all the **Ingredients:** except the cooking spray, stir well and shape medium cakes out of this mixture
Place the cakes in your air fryer's basket, grease them with cooking spray and cook at 380°F for 6 minutes on each side. Serve as an appetizer.
Nutrition: Calories: 165; Fat: 5g; Fiber: 2g; Carbs: 3g; Protein: 7g

Tomato Bites

Preparation Time: 25 minutes
Servings: 6
Ingredients:
6 tomatoes; halved
2 oz. watercress

3 oz. cheddar cheese; grated
1 tbsp. olive oil
3 tsp. sugar-free apricot jam
2 tsp. oregano; dried
A pinch of salt and black pepper

Directions:

Spread the jam on each tomato half, sprinkle oregano, salt and pepper and drizzle the oil all over them

Introduce them in the fryer's basket, sprinkle the cheese on top and cook at 360°F for 20 minutes

Arrange the tomatoes on a platter, top each half with some watercress and serve as an appetizer.

Nutrition: Calories: 131; Fat: 7g; Fiber: 2g; Carbs: 4g; Protein: 7g

Spinach Rolls

Preparation Time: 26 minutes
Servings: 6
Ingredients:

3 cups mozzarella; shredded
6 oz. spinach; chopped.
4 oz. cream cheese, soft
½ cup almond flour
2 eggs; whisked
¼ cup parmesan; grated
2 tbsp. ghee; melted
4 tbsp. coconut flour
A pinch of salt and black pepper

Directions:

Take a bowl and mix the mozzarella with coconut and almond flour, eggs, salt and pepper, stir well until you obtain a dough and roll it well on a parchment paper

Cut into triangles and leave them aside for now

Take a bowl and mix the spinach with parmesan, cream cheese, salt and pepper and stir really well.

Divide this into the center of each dough triangle, roll and seal the edges

Brush the rolls with the ghee, place them in your air fryer's basket and cook at 360°F for 20 minutes. Serve as an appetizer.

Nutrition: Calories: 210; Fat: 8g; Fiber: 1g; Carbs: 3g; Protein: 8g

Green Beans Snack

Preparation Time: 17 minutes
Servings: 4
Ingredients:

12 oz. green beans; trimmed
1 egg; whisked
1 cup parmesan; grated
¼ tsp. sweet paprika
A pinch of salt and black pepper

Directions:

Take a bowl and mix the parmesan with salt, pepper and the paprika and stir.

Put the egg in a separate bowl, Dredge the green beans in egg and then in the parmesan mix

Arrange the green beans in your air fryer's basket and cook at 380°F for 12 minutes.

Nutrition: Calories: 112; Fat: 6g; Fiber: 1g; Carbs: 2g; Protein: 9g

Brussels Sprouts Wraps

Preparation Time: 25 minutes
Servings: 12
Ingredients:
12 Brussels sprouts
12 bacon strips
A drizzle of olive oil
Directions:
Wrap each Brussels sprouts in a bacon strip, brush them with some oil.
Put them in your air fryer's basket and cook at 350°F for 20 minutes
Nutrition: Calories: 140; Fat: 5g; Fiber: 2g; Carbs: 4g; Protein: 4g

Pickled Snack

Preparation Time: 25 minutes
Servings: 4
Ingredients:
4 dill pickle spears; sliced in half and quartered
1 cup avocado mayonnaise
8 bacon slices; halved
Directions:
Wrap each pickle spear in a bacon slice, put them in your air fryer's basket and cook at 400°F for 20 minutes.
Serve as a snack with the mayonnaise
Nutrition: Calories: 100; Fat: 4g; Fiber: 2g; Carbs: 3g; Protein: 4g

Avocado Wraps

Preparation Time: 20 minutes
Servings: 4
Ingredients:
2 avocados, peeled, pitted and cut into 12 wedges
1 tbsp. ghee; melted
12 bacon strips
Directions:
Wrap each avocado wedge in a bacon strip, brush them with the ghee.
Put them in your air fryer's basket and cook at 360°F for 15 minutes. Serve as an appetizer
Nutrition: Calories: 161; Fat: 4g; Fiber: 2g; Carbs: 4g; Protein: 6g

Chicken Party Meatballs

Preparation Time: 25 minutes
Servings: 12
Ingredients:
2 lb. chicken breast, skinless; boneless and ground
2 garlic cloves; minced
2 spring onions; chopped.
¾ cup almond meal
6 tbsp. hot sauce
2 tbsp. ghee; melted
Cooking spray
A pinch of salt and black pepper

Directions:

Take a bowl and mix all the **Ingredients:** except the cooking spray, stir well and shape medium meatballs out of this mix

Arrange the meatballs in your air fryer's basket, grease them with cooking spray and cook at 360°F for 20 minutes.

Nutrition: Calories: 257; Fat: 14g; Fiber: 1g; Carbs: 3g; Protein: 17g

Cucumber Salsa

Preparation Time: 10 minutes

Servings: 4

Ingredients:

1 ½ lb. cucumbers; sliced

2 red chili peppers; chopped.

2 tomatoes cubed

2 spring onions; chopped.

1 tbsp. balsamic vinegar

2 tbsp. ginger; grated

A drizzle of olive oil

Directions:

In a pan that fits your air fryer, mix all the **Ingredients:**, toss, introduce in the fryer and cook at 340°F for 5 minutes

Divide into bowls and serve cold as an appetizer.

Nutrition: Calories: 150; Fat: 2g; Fiber: 1g; Carbs: 2g; Protein: 4g

Parsley Meatballs

Preparation Time: 25 minutes

Servings: 6

Ingredients:

1 lb. beef meat, ground

2 tbsp. parsley; chopped.

1 tsp. onion powder

1 tsp. garlic powder

Cooking spray

A pinch of salt and black pepper

Directions:

Take a bowl and mix all the **Ingredients:** except the cooking spray, stir well and shape medium meatballs out of this mix

Pace them in your lined air fryer's basket, grease with cooking spray and cook at 360°F for 20 minutes

Nutrition: Calories: 180; Fat: 5g; Fiber: 2g; Carbs: 5g; Protein: 7g

Radish Chips

Preparation Time: 20 minutes

Servings: 4

Ingredients:

16 oz. radishes, thinly sliced

2 tbsp. coconut oil; melted

A pinch of salt and black pepper

Directions:

Take a bowl and mix the radish slices with salt, pepper and the oil, toss well, place them in your air fryer's basket and cook at 400°F for 15 minutes, flipping them halfway

Nutrition: Calories: 174; Fat: 5g; Fiber: 1g; Carbs: 3g; Protein: 6g

Pork Belly Bites

Preparation Time: 35 minutes
Servings: 6
Ingredients:
2 lb. pork belly; cut into strips
2 tbsp. olive oil
A pinch of salt and black pepper
A pinch of basil; dried
2 tsp. fennel seeds
Directions:
Take a bowl and mix all the **Ingredients:**, toss and put the pork strips in your air fryer's basket and cook at 425°F for 25 minutes
Divide into bowls and serve as a snack.
Nutrition: Calories: 251; Fat: 14g; Fiber: 3g; Carbs: 5g; Protein: 18g

Olives Dip

Preparation Time: 10 minutes
Servings: 6
Ingredients:
1 cup black olives, pitted and chopped.
¼ cup capers
½ cup olive oil
1 cup parsley leaves
1 cup basil leaves
2 garlic cloves; minced
3 tbsp. lemon juice
2 tsp. apple cider vinegar
A pinch of salt and black pepper
Directions:
In a blender, combine all the **Ingredients:**, pulse well and transfer to a ramekin.
Place the ramekin in your air fryer's basket and cook at 350°F for 5 minutes
Nutrition: Calories: 120; Fat: 5g; Fiber: 2g; Carbs: 3g; Protein: 7g

Salmon Spread

Preparation Time: 11 minutes
Servings: 4
Ingredients:
8 oz. cream cheese, soft
½ cup coconut cream
4 oz. smoked salmon, skinless; boneless and minced
2 tbsp. lemon juice
1 tbsp. chives; chopped.
A pinch of salt and black pepper
Directions:
Take a bowl and mix all the **Ingredients:** and whisk them really well.
Transfer the mix to a ramekin, place it in your air fryer's basket and cook at 360°F for 6 minutes
Nutrition: Calories: 180; Fat: 7g; Fiber: 1g; Carbs: 5g; Protein: 7g

Shrimp Snack

Preparation Time: 15 minutes
Servings: 4
Ingredients:
1 lb. shrimp; peeled and deveined
¼ cup olive oil
3 garlic cloves; minced
¼ tsp. cayenne pepper
Juice of ½ lemon
A pinch of salt and black pepper
Directions:
In a pan that fits your air fryer, mix all the **Ingredients:**, toss,
Introduce in the fryer and cook at 370°F for 10 minutes. Serve as a snack
Nutrition: Calories: 242; Fat: 14g; Fiber: 2g; Carbs: 3g; Protein: 17g

Pork Rind Nachos

Preparation Time: 10 minutes
Servings: 2
Ingredients:
1 oz. pork rinds.
4 oz. shredded cooked chicken.
¼ cup guacamole.
½ cup shredded Monterey jack cheese.
¼ cup full-fat sour cream.
¼ cup sliced pickled jalapeños.
Directions:
Place pork rinds into 6-inch round baking pan. Cover with shredded chicken and Monterey jack cheese. Place pan into the air fryer basket.
Adjust the temperature to 370 Degrees F and set the timer for 5 minutes or until cheese is melted.
Top with jalapeños, guacamole and sour cream. Serve immediately.
Nutrition: Calories: 395; Protein: 31g; Fiber: 2g; Fat: 25g; Carbs: 0g

Avocado Balls

Preparation Time: 10 minutes
Servings: 4
Ingredients:
1 avocado, peeled, pitted and mashed
4 bacon slices, cooked and crumbled
2 spring onions; minced
1 chili pepper; chopped.
¼ cup ghee; melted
2 garlic cloves; minced
2 tbsp. cilantro
1 tbsp. lime juice
A pinch of salt and black pepper
Cooking spray
Directions:
Take a bowl and mix all the **Ingredients:** except the cooking spray, stir well and shape medium balls out of this mix
Place them in your air fryer's basket, grease with cooking spray and cook at 370°F for 5 minutes.

Nutrition: Calories: 160; Fat: 6g; Fiber: 3g; Carbs: 4g; Protein: 6g

Spinach Rolls

Preparation Time: 26 minutes
Servings: 6
Ingredients:
3 cups mozzarella; shredded
6 oz. spinach; chopped.
4 oz. cream cheese, soft
½ cup almond flour
2 eggs; whisked
¼ cup parmesan; grated
2 tbsp. ghee; melted
4 tbsp. coconut flour
A pinch of salt and black pepper
Directions:
Take a bowl and mix the mozzarella with coconut and almond flour, eggs, salt and pepper, stir well until you obtain a dough and roll it well on a parchment paper
Cut into triangles and leave them aside for now
Take a bowl and mix the spinach with parmesan, cream cheese, salt and pepper and stir really well.
Divide this into the center of each dough triangle, roll and seal the edges
Brush the rolls with the ghee, place them in your air fryer's basket and cook at 360°F for 20 minutes. Serve as an appetizer.
Nutrition: Calories: 210; Fat: 8g; Fiber: 1g; Carbs: 3g; Protein: 8g

Smoked Salmon Bites

Preparation Time: 15 minutes
Servings: 12
Ingredients:
4 oz. smoked salmon, skinless; boneless and chopped.
2 avocados, peeled, pitted and mashed
2 tbsp. coconut cream
1 tsp. dill; chopped.
1 tsp. avocado oil
A pinch of salt and black pepper
Directions:
Take a bowl and mix all the **Ingredients:**, stir well and shape medium balls out of this mix.
Place them in your air fryer's basket and cook at 350°F for 10 minutes
Nutrition: Calories: 100; Fat: 2g; Fiber: 1g; Carbs: 2g; Protein: 2g

Chili Meatballs

Preparation Time: 25 minutes
Servings: 12
Ingredients:
1 lb. pork meat, ground
3 spring onions; minced
2 garlic cloves; minced
1 chili pepper; minced
3 tbsp. cilantro; chopped.
1 tbsp. ginger; grated

1 ½ tbsp. coconut aminos
A pinch of salt and black pepper
Cooking spray

Directions:

Take a bowl and mix all the **Ingredients:** except the cooking spray, stir really well and shape medium meatballs out of this mix

Arrange them in your air fryer's basket, grease with cooking spray and cook at 380°F for 20 minutes.

Nutrition: Calories: 200; Fat: 12g; Fiber: 2g; Carbs: 3g; Protein: 14g

Mushroom Platter

Preparation Time: 17 minutes
Servings: 4
Ingredients:

12 oz. Portobello mushrooms; sliced
2 tbsp. olive oil
2 tbsp. balsamic vinegar
½ tsp. rosemary; dried
½ tsp. thyme; dried
½ tsp. basil; dried
½ tsp. tarragon; dried
A pinch of salt and black pepper

Directions:

Take a bowl and mix all the **Ingredients:** and toss well.

Arrange the mushroom slices in your air fryer's basket and cook at 380°F for 12 minutes. Arrange the mushroom slices on a platter and serve

Nutrition: Calories: 147; Fat: 8g; Fiber: 2g; Carbs: 3g; Protein: 3g

Asparagus Wraps

Preparation Time: 20 minutes
Servings: 8
Ingredients:

16 asparagus spears; trimmed
16 bacon strips
1 tbsp. lemon juice
2 tbsp. olive oil
1 tsp. oregano; chopped.
1 tsp. thyme; chopped.
A pinch of salt and black pepper

Directions:

Take a bowl and mix the oil with lemon juice, the herbs, salt and pepper and whisk well.

Brush the asparagus spears with this mix and wrap each in a bacon strip

Arrange the asparagus wraps in your air fryer's basket and cook at 390°F for 15 minutes.

Nutrition: Calories: 173; Fat: 4g; Fiber: 2g; Carbs: 3g; Protein: 6g

Spinach Artichoke Dip

Preparation Time: 20 minutes
Servings: 6
Ingredients:

10 oz. frozen spinach, drained and thawed
8 oz. full-fat cream cheese; softened.

1 (14-oz.can artichoke hearts, drained and chopped
1/4 cup chopped pickled jalapeños.
1/4 cup full-fat mayonnaise
1/4 cup full-fat sour cream.
1/4 cup grated Parmesan cheese.
1 cup shredded pepper jack cheese
1/2 tsp. garlic powder.
Directions:
Mix all **Ingredients:** in a 4-cup baking bowl. Place into the air fryer basket.
Adjust the temperature to 320 Degrees F and set the timer for 10 minutes. Remove when brown and bubbling. Serve warm.
Nutrition: Calories: 226; Protein: 10g; Fiber: 7g; Fat: 19g; Carbs: 12g

Spinach and Onion Dip

Preparation Time: 25 minutes
Servings: 6
Ingredients:
1 lb. spinach; torn
1 cup mozzarella; shredded
1 cup coconut cream
4 spring onions; chopped.
6 tbsp. ghee; melted
Salt and black pepper to taste.
Directions:
In a pan that fits the air fryer, combine all the **Ingredients:** and whisk them really well.
Introduce the pan in your air fryer and cook at 370°F for 20 minutes. Divide into bowls and serve
Nutrition: Calories: 184; Fat: 12g; Fiber: 2g; Carbs: 3g; Protein: 9g

Cheddar Dip

Preparation Time: 17 minutes
Servings: 6
Ingredients:
8 oz. cheddar cheese; grated
12 oz. coconut cream
2 tsp. hot sauce
Directions:
In ramekin, mix the cream with hot sauce and cheese and whisk.
Put the ramekin in the fryer and cook at 390°F for 12 minutes. Whisk, divide into bowls and serve as a dip
Nutrition: Calories: 170; Fat: 9g; Fiber: 2g; Carbs: 4g; Protein: 12g

Turkey and Cheese Balls

Preparation Time: 25 minutes
Servings: 8
Ingredients:
1 lb. turkey breast, skinless; boneless and ground
1/2 cup parmesan; grated
1/2 cup coconut milk
2 cups mozzarella; grated
1/2 cup almond meal
1 tbsp. Italian seasoning

3 tbsp. ghee; melted
1 tsp. garlic powder
Cooking spray

Directions:

Take a bowl and mix all the **Ingredients:** except the parmesan and the cooking spray and stir well.

Shape medium balls out of this mix, coat each in the parmesan and arrange them in your air fryer

Grease the balls with cooking spray and cook at 380°F for 20 minutes.

Nutrition: Calories: 210; Fat: 12g; Fiber: 2g; Carbs: 4g; Protein: 14g

Wrapped Parmesan Asparagus

Preparation Time: 20 minutes
Servings: 4
Ingredients:

1 lb. asparagus
12 (5-oz.slices prosciutto
⅓ cup grated Parmesan cheese.
1 tbsp. coconut oil; melted
2 tbsp. salted butter; melted.
⅛ tsp. red pepper flakes
2 tsp. lemon juice

Directions:

On a clean work surface, place an asparagus spear onto a slice of prosciutto

Drizzle with coconut oil and lemon juice. Sprinkle red pepper flakes and Parmesan across asparagus. Roll prosciutto around asparagus spear. Place into the air fryer basket

Adjust the temperature to 375 Degrees F and set the timer for 10 minutes. Drizzle the asparagus roll with butter before serving.

Nutrition: Calories: 263; Protein: 19g; Fiber: 4g; Fat: 22g; Carbs: 7g

Cilantro Dip

Preparation Time: 13 minutes
Servings: 6
Ingredients:

½ cup cashews, soaked in water for 4 hours and drained
2 garlic cloves; minced
2 tbsp. coconut milk
3 tbsp. cilantro; chopped.
1 tsp. lime juice
A pinch of salt and black pepper

Directions:

In a blender, combine all the **Ingredients:**, pulse well and transfer to a ramekin.

Put the ramekin in your air fryer's basket and cook at 350°F for 8 minutes. Serve as a dip

Nutrition: Calories: 144; Fat: 2g; Fiber: 1g; Carbs: 3g; Protein: 4g

Tuna Appetizer

Preparation Time: 15 minutes
Servings: 2
Ingredients:

1 lb. tuna, skinless; boneless and cubed
3 scallion stalks; minced

1 chili pepper; minced
2 tomatoes; cubed
1 tbsp. coconut aminos
2 tbsp. olive oil
1 tbsp. coconut cream
1 tsp. sesame seeds

Directions:

In a pan that fits your air fryer, mix all the **Ingredients:** except the sesame seeds, toss, introduce in the fryer and cook at 360°F for 10 minutes

Divide into bowls and serve as an appetizer with sesame seeds sprinkled on top.

Nutrition: Calories: 231; Fat: 18g; Fiber: 3g; Carbs: 4g; Protein: 18g

Tomato Bites

Preparation Time: 25 minutes
Servings: 6
Ingredients:

6 tomatoes; halved
2 oz. watercress
3 oz. cheddar cheese; grated
1 tbsp. olive oil
3 tsp. sugar-free apricot jam
2 tsp. oregano; dried
A pinch of salt and black pepper

Directions:

Spread the jam on each tomato half, sprinkle oregano, salt and pepper and drizzle the oil all over them

Introduce them in the fryer's basket, sprinkle the cheese on top and cook at 360°F for 20 minutes

Arrange the tomatoes on a platter, top each half with some watercress and serve as an appetizer.

Nutrition: Calories: 131; Fat: 7g; Fiber: 2g; Carbs: 4g; Protein: 7g

Tomatoes Dip

Preparation Time: 25 minutes
Servings: 6
Ingredients:

12 oz. cream cheese, soft
8 oz. mozzarella cheese; grated
¼ cup basil; chopped.
¼ cup parmesan; grated
4 garlic cloves; minced
1 pint grape tomatoes; halved
2 tbsp. thyme; chopped.
½ tbsp. oregano; chopped.
1 tsp. olive oil
A pinch of salt and black pepper

Directions:

Put the tomatoes in your air fryer's basket and cook them at 400°F for 15 minutes.

In a blender, combine the fried tomatoes with the rest of the **Ingredients:** and pulse well

Transfer this to a ramekin, place it in the air fryer and cook at 400°F for 5 - 6 minutes more.

Serve as a snack

Nutrition: Calories: 184; Fat: 8g; Fiber: 3g; Carbs: 4g; Protein: 8g

Artichokes Dip

Preparation Time: 30 minutes
Servings: 6
Ingredients:
2 garlic cloves; minced
6 oz. cream cheese, soft
½ cup almond milk
2 spring onions; minced
20 oz. canned artichoke hearts, drained and chopped.
1 cup mozzarella; shredded
2 tsp. olive oil
A pinch of salt and black pepper
Directions:
Grease a baking pan that fits the air fryer with the oil and mix all the **Ingredients:** except the mozzarella inside.
Sprinkle the cheese all over, introduce the pan in the air fryer and cook at 370°F for 25 minutes
Divide into bowls and serve as a party dip
Nutrition: Calories: 231; Fat: 11g; Fiber: 2g; Carbs: 4g; Protein: 8g

BBQ Roasted Almonds

Preparation Time: 11 minutes
Servings: 4
Ingredients:
1 cup raw almonds
¼ tsp. smoked paprika
¼ tsp. onion powder.
¼ tsp. cumin
2 tsp. coconut oil
1 tsp. chili powder
Directions:
Take a large bowl, toss all **Ingredients:** until almonds are evenly coated with oil and spices. Place almonds into the air fryer basket
Adjust the temperature to 320 Degrees F and set the timer for 6 minutes. Toss the fryer basket halfway through the cooking time. Allow to cool completely.
Nutrition: Calories: 182; Protein: 2g; Fiber: 3g; Fat: 13g; Carbs: 6g

Baby Carrots with Asian Flair

Preparation Time: 20 minutes
Servings: 3
Nutrition: 165 Calories; 3g Fat; 26g Carbs; 6g Protein; 18g Sugars
Ingredients:
1 pound baby carrots
2 tablespoons sesame oil
1/2 teaspoon Szechuan pepper
1 teaspoon Wuxiang powder (Five-spice powder
1 tablespoon honey
1 large garlic clove, crushed
1 (1-inchpiece fresh ginger root, peeled and grated
2 tablespoons tamari sauce

Directions:
Start by preheating your Air Fryer to 380 degrees F.
Toss all **Ingredients:** together and place them in the Air Fryer basket.
Cook for 15 minutes, shaking the basket halfway through the cooking time. Enjoy!

Mexican-Style Corn on the Cob with Bacon

Preparation Time: 20 minutes
Servings: 4
Nutrition: 261 Calories; 12g Fat; 35g Carbs; 4g Protein; 1g Sugars
Ingredients:
2 slices bacon
4 ears fresh corn, shucked and cut into halves
1 avocado, pitted, peeled and mashed
1 teaspoon ancho chili powder
2 garlic cloves
2 tablespoons cilantro, chopped
1 teaspoon lime juice
Salt and black pepper, to taste
Directions:
Start by preheating your Air Fryer to 400 degrees F. Cook the bacon for 6 to 7 minutes; chop into small chunks and reserve.
Spritz the corn with cooking spray. Cook at 395 degrees F for 8 minutes, turning them over halfway through the cooking time.
Mix the reserved bacon with the remaining **Ingredients:**. Spoon the bacon mixture over the corn on the cob and serve immediately. Bon appétit!

Beer Battered Vidalia Rings

Preparation Time: 30 minutes
Servings: 4
Nutrition: 318 Calories; 17g Fat; 49g Carbs; 4g Protein; 2g Sugars
Ingredients:
1/2 pound Vidalia onions, sliced into rings
1/2 cup all-purpose flour
1/4 cup cornmeal
1/2 teaspoon baking powder
Sea salt and freshly cracked black pepper, to taste
1/4 teaspoon garlic powder
2 eggs, beaten
1/2 cup lager-style beer
1 cup plain breadcrumbs
2 tablespoons peanut oil
Directions:
Place the onion rings in the bowl with icy cold water; let them soak approximately 20 minutes; drain the onion rings and pat them dry.
In a shallow bowl, mix the flour, cornmeal, baking powder, salt, and black pepper. Add the garlic powder, eggs and beer; mix well to combine.
In another shallow bowl, mix the breadcrumbs with the peanut oil. Dip the onion rings in the flour/egg mixture; then, dredge in the breadcrumb mixture. Roll to coat them evenly.
Spritz the Air Fryer basket with cooking spray; arrange the breaded onion rings in the basket.
Cook in the preheated Air Fryer at 400 degrees F for 4 to 5 minutes, turning them over halfway through the cooking time. Bon appétit!

Wonton Sausage Appetizers

Preparation Time: 20 minutes
Servings: 5
Nutrition: 199 Calories; 8g Fat; 12g Carbs; 14g Protein; 3g Sugars
Ingredients:
1/2 pound ground sausage
2 tablespoons scallions, chopped
1 garlic clove, minced
1/2 tablespoon fish sauce
1 teaspoon Sriracha sauce
20 wonton wrappers
1 egg, whisked with 1 tablespoon water
Directions:
In a mixing bowl, thoroughly combine the ground sausage, scallions, garlic, fish sauce, and Sriracha.
Divide the mixture between the wonton wrappers. Dip your fingers in the egg wash
Fold the wonton in half. Bring up the 2 ends of the wonton and use the egg wash to stick them together. Pinch the edges and coat each wonton with the egg wash.
Place the folded wontons in the lightly greased cooking basket. Cook at 360 degrees F for 10 minutes. Work in batches and serve warm. Bon appétit!

Cocktail Cranberry Meatballs

Preparation Time: 15 minutes
Servings: 5
Nutrition: 365 Calories; 16g Fat; 31g Carbs; 26g Protein; 24g Sugars
Ingredients:
1/2 pound ground beef
1/2 pound ground turkey
1/4 cup Parmesan cheese, grated
1/4 cup breadcrumbs
1 small shallot, chopped
2 eggs, whisked
1/2 teaspoon garlic powder
1/2 teaspoon porcini powder
Sea salt and ground black pepper, to taste
1 teaspoon red pepper flakes, crushed
1 tablespoon soy sauce
1 (8-ouncecan jellied cranberry sauce
6 ounces tomato-based chili sauce
Directions:
In a mixing bowl, combine the ground meat together with the cheese, breadcrumbs, shallot, eggs, and spices.
Shape the mixture into 1-inch balls.
Cook the meatballs in the preheated Air Fryer at 380 degrees for 5 minutes. Shake halfway through the cooking time. Work in batches.
Whisk the soy sauce, cranberry sauce, and chili sauce in a mixing bowl. Pour the sauce over the meatballs and bake an additional 2 minutes.
Serve with cocktail sticks. Bon appétit!

Paprika Potato Chips

Preparation Time: 50 minutes
Servings: 3
Nutrition: 190 Calories; 3g Fat; 48g Carbs; 7g Protein; 1g Sugars
Ingredients:
3 potatoes, thinly sliced
1 teaspoon sea salt
1 teaspoon garlic powder
1 teaspoon paprika
1/4 cup ketchup
Directions:
Add the sliced potatoes to a bowl with salted water. Let them soak for 30 minutes. Drain and rinse your potatoes.
Pat dry and toss with salt.
Cook in the preheated Air Fryer at 400 degrees F for 15 minutes, shaking the basket occasionally. Work in batches. Toss with the garlic powder and paprika. Serve with ketchup. Enjoy!

Barbecue Little Smokies

Preparation Time: 20 minutes
Servings: 6
Nutrition: 182 Calories; 6g Fat; 12g Carbs; 19g Protein; 17g Sugars
Ingredients:
1 pound beef cocktail wieners
10 ounces barbecue sauce
Directions:
Start by preheating your Air Fryer to 380 degrees F.
Prick holes into your sausages using a fork and transfer them to the baking pan.
Cook for 13 minutes. Spoon the barbecue sauce into the pan and cook an additional 2 minutes. Serve with toothpicks. Bon appétit!

Sweet Potato Fries with Spicy Dip

Preparation Time: 50 minutes
Servings: 3
Nutrition: 332 Calories; 26g Fat; 29g Carbs; 3g Protein; 8g Sugars
Ingredients:
3 medium sweet potatoes, cut into 1/3-inch sticks
2 tablespoons olive oil
1 teaspoon kosher salt
Spicy Dip:
1/4 cup mayonnaise
1/4 cup Greek yogurt
1/4 teaspoon Dijon mustard
1 teaspoon hot sauce
Directions:
Soak the sweet potato in icy cold water for 30 minutes. Drain the sweet potatoes and pat them dry with paper towels.
Toss the sweet potatoes with olive oil and salt.
Place in the lightly greased cooking basket. Cook in the preheated Air Fryer at 360 degrees F for 14 minutes. Wok in batches.

While the sweet potatoes are cooking, make the spicy dip by whisking the remaining **Ingredients:**. Place in the refrigerator until ready to serve. Enjoy!

Crunchy Broccoli Fries

Preparation Time: 15 minutes
Servings: 4
Nutrition: 127 Calories; 6g Fat; 9g Carbs; 9g Protein; 6g Sugars
Ingredients:
1 pound broccoli florets
1/2 teaspoon onion powder
1 teaspoon granulated garlic
1/2 teaspoon cayenne pepper
Sea salt and ground black pepper, to taste
2 tablespoons sesame oil
4 tablespoons parmesan cheese, preferably freshly grated
Directions:
Start by preheating the Air Fryer to 400 degrees F.
Blanch the broccoli in salted boiling water until al dente, about 3 to 4 minutes. Drain well and transfer to the lightly greased Air Fryer basket.
Add the onion powder, garlic, cayenne pepper, salt, black pepper, and sesame oil.
Cook for 6 minutes, tossing halfway through the cooking time. Bon appétit!

Kale Chips with Tahini Sauce

Preparation Time: 15 minutes
Servings: 4
Nutrition: 170 Calories; 15g Fat; 1g Carbs; 2g Protein; 7g Sugars
Ingredients:
5 cups kale leaves, torn into 1-inch pieces
1 ½ tablespoons sesame oil
1/2 teaspoon shallot powder
1 teaspoon garlic powder
1/4 teaspoon porcini powder
1/2 teaspoon mustard seeds
1 teaspoon salt
1/3 cup tahini (sesame butter
1 tablespoon fresh lemon juice
2 cloves garlic, minced
Directions:
Toss the kale with the sesame oil and seasonings.
Bake in the preheated Air Fryer at 350 degrees F for 10 minutes, shaking the cooking basket occasionally.
Bake until the edges are brown. Work in batches.
Meanwhile, make the sauce by whisking all **Ingredients:** in a small mixing bowl. Serve and enjoy!

Famous Blooming Onion with Mayo Dip

Preparation Time: 25 minutes
Servings: 3
Nutrition: 222 Calories; 9g Fat; 26g Carbs; 6g Protein; 9g Sugars
Ingredients:
1 large Vidalia onion

1/2 cup all-purpose flour
1 teaspoon salt
1/2 teaspoon ground black pepper
1 teaspoon cayenne pepper
1/2 teaspoon dried thyme
1/2 teaspoon dried oregano
1/2 teaspoon ground cumin
2 eggs
1/4 cup milk
Mayo Dip:
3 tablespoons mayonnaise
3 tablespoons sour cream
1 tablespoon horseradish, drained
Kosher salt and freshly ground black pepper, to taste
Directions:
Cut off the top 1/2 inch of the Vidalia onion; peel your onion and place it cut-side down. Starting 1/2 inch from the root, cut the onion in half. Make a second cut that splits each half in two. You will have 4 quarters held together by the root.
Repeat these cuts, splitting the 4 quarters to yield eighths; then, you should split them again until you have 16 evenly spaced cuts. Turn the onion over and gently separate the outer pieces using your fingers.
In a mixing bowl, thoroughly combine the flour and spices. In a separate bowl, whisk the eggs and milk. Dip the onion into the egg mixture, followed by the flour mixture.
Spritz the onion with cooking spray and transfer to the lightly greased cooking basket. Cook for 370 degrees F for 12 to 15 minutes.
Meanwhile, make the mayo dip by whisking the remaining **Ingredients:**. Serve and enjoy!

Thyme-Roasted Sweet Potatoes

Preparation Time: 35 minutes
Servings: 3
Nutrition: 143 Calories; 7g Fat; 13g Carbs; 7g Protein; 0g Sugars
Ingredients:
1 pound sweet potatoes, peeled, cut into bite-sized pieces
2 tablespoons olive oil
1 teaspoon sea salt
1/4 teaspoon freshly ground black pepper
1/2 teaspoon cayenne pepper
2 fresh thyme sprigs
Directions:
Arrange the potato slices in a single layer in the lightly greased cooking basket. Add the olive oil, salt, black pepper, and cayenne pepper; toss to coat.
Bake at 380 degrees F for 30 minutes, shaking the cooking basket occasionally.
Bake until tender and slightly browned, working in batches. Serve warm, garnished with thyme sprigs. Bon appétit!

Chicken Nuggets with Campfire Sauce

Preparation Time: 20 minutes
Servings: 6
Nutrition: 211 Calories; 4g Fat; 14g Carbs; 19g Protein; 3g Sugars
Ingredients:
1 pound chicken breasts, slice into tenders

1/2 teaspoon cayenne pepper
Salt and black pepper, to taste
1/4 cup cornmeal
1 egg, whisked
1/2 cup seasoned breadcrumbs
1/4 cup mayo
1/4 cup barbecue sauce

Directions:

Pat the chicken tenders dry with a kitchen towel. Season with the cayenne pepper, salt, and black pepper.

Dip the chicken tenders into the cornmeal, followed by the egg. Press the chicken tenders into the breadcrumbs, coating evenly.

Place the chicken tenders in the lightly greased Air Fryer basket. Cook at 360 degrees for 9 to 12 minutes, turning them over to cook evenly.

In a mixing bowl, thoroughly combine the mayonnaise with the barbecue sauce. Serve the chicken nuggets with the sauce for dipping. Bon appétit!

Avocado Fries with Chipotle Sauce

Preparation Time: 20 minutes
Servings: 3
Nutrition: 273 Calories; 14g Fat; 21g Carbs; 7g Protein; 7g Sugars
Ingredients:

2 tablespoons fresh lime juice
1 avocado, pitted, peeled, and sliced
Pink Himalayan salt and ground white pepper, to taste
1/4 cup flour
1 egg
1/2 cup breadcrumbs
1 chipotle chili in adobo sauce
1/4 cup light mayonnaise
1/4 cup plain Greek yogurt

Directions:

Drizzle lime juice all over the avocado slices and set aside.

Then, set up your breading station. Mix the salt, pepper, and all-purpose flour in a shallow dish. In a separate dish, whisk the egg.

Finally, place your breadcrumbs in a third dish.

Start by dredging the avocado slices in the flour mixture; then, dip them into the egg. Press the avocado slices into the breadcrumbs, coating evenly.

Cook in the preheating Air Fryer at 380 degrees F for 11 minutes, shaking the cooking basket halfway through the cooking time.

Meanwhile, blend the chipotle chili, mayo, and Greek yogurt in your food processor until the sauce is creamy and uniform.

Serve the warm avocado slices with the sauce on the side. Enjoy!

Asian Twist Chicken Wings

Preparation Time: 20 minutes
Servings: 6
Nutrition: 195 Calories; 7g Fat; 4g Carbs; 25g Protein; 4g Sugars
Ingredients:

1 ½ pounds chicken wings
2 teaspoons sesame oil

Kosher salt and ground black pepper, to taste
2 tablespoons tamari sauce
1 tablespoon rice vinegar
2 garlic clove, minced
2 tablespoons honey
2 sun-dried tomatoes, minced

Directions:

Toss the chicken wings with the sesame oil, salt, and pepper. Add chicken wings to a lightly greased baking pan.

Roast the chicken wings in the preheated Air Fryer at 390 degrees F for 7 minutes. Turn them over once or twice to ensure even cooking.

In a mixing dish, thoroughly combine the tamari sauce, vinegar, garlic, honey, and sun-dried tomatoes.

Pour the sauce all over the chicken wings; bake an additional 5 minutes. Bon appétit!

Roasted Cauliflower Florets

Preparation Time: 20 minutes
Servings: 2
Nutrition: 80 Calories; 9g Fat; 9g Carbs; 1g Protein; 1g Sugars
Ingredients:
3 cups cauliflower florets
2 teaspoons sesame oil
1 teaspoon onion powder
1 teaspoon garlic powder
Sea salt and cracked black pepper, to taste
1 teaspoon paprika

Directions:

Start by preheating your Air Fryer to 400 degrees F.

Toss the cauliflower with the remaining **Ingredients:**; toss to coat well.

Cook for 12 minutes, shaking the cooking basket halfway through the cooking time. They will crisp up as they cool. Bon appétit!

Parsnip Chips with Spicy Citrus Aioli

Preparation Time: 20 minutes
Servings: 4
Nutrition: 207 Calories; 11g Fat; 28g Carbs; 8g Protein; 7g Sugars
Ingredients:
1 pound parsnips, peel long strips
2 tablespoons sesame oil
Sea salt and ground black pepper, to taste
1 teaspoon red pepper flakes, crushed
1/2 teaspoon curry powder
1/2 teaspoon mustard seeds
Spicy Citrus Aioli:
1/4 cup mayonnaise
1 tablespoon fresh lime juice
1 clove garlic, smashed
Salt and black pepper, to taste

Directions:

Start by preheating the Air Fryer to 380 degrees F.

Toss the parsnip chips with the sesame oil, salt, black pepper, red pepper, curry powder, and mustard seeds.

Cook for 15 minutes, shaking the Air Fryer basket periodically.

Meanwhile, make the sauce by whisking the mayonnaise, lime juice, garlic, salt, and pepper. Place in the refrigerator until ready to use. Bon appétit!

Classic Deviled Eggs

Preparation Time: 20 minutes
Servings: 3
Nutrition: 261 Calories; 12g Fat; 5g Carbs; 15g Protein; 1g Sugars
Ingredients:

5 eggs
2 tablespoons mayonnaise
2 tablespoons sweet pickle relish
Sea salt, to taste
1/2 teaspoon mixed peppercorns, crushed

Directions:

Place the wire rack in the Air Fryer basket; lower the eggs onto the wire rack.

Cook at 270 degrees F for 15 minutes.

Transfer them to an ice-cold water bath to stop the cooking. Peel the eggs under cold running water; slice them into halves.

Mash the egg yolks with the mayo, sweet pickle relish, and salt; spoon yolk mixture into egg whites. Arrange on a nice serving platter and garnish with the mixed peppercorns. Bon appétit!

Cajun Cheese Sticks

Preparation Time: 15 minutes
Servings: 4
Nutrition: 372 Calories; 27g Fat; 15g Carbs; 28g Protein; 8g Sugars
Ingredients:

1/2 cup all-purpose flour
2 eggs
1/2 cup parmesan cheese, grated
1 tablespoon Cajun seasonings
8 cheese sticks, kid-friendly
1/4 cup ketchup

Directions:

To begin, set up your breading station. Place the all-purpose flour in a shallow dish. In a separate dish, whisk the eggs.

Finally, mix the parmesan cheese and Cajun seasoning in a third dish.

Start by dredging the cheese sticks in the flour; then, dip them into the egg. Press the cheese sticks into the parmesan mixture, coating evenly.

Place the breaded cheese sticks in the lightly greased Air Fryer basket. Cook at 380 degrees F for 6 minutes.

Serve with ketchup and enjoy!

Puerto Rican Tostones

Preparation Time: 15 minutes
Servings: 2
Nutrition: 151 Calories; 1g Fat; 29g Carbs; 6g Protein; 17g Sugars
Ingredients:

1 ripe plantain, sliced

1 tablespoon sunflower oil
A pinch of grated nutmeg
A pinch of kosher salt
Directions:
Toss the plantains with the oil, nutmeg, and salt in a bowl.
Cook in the preheated Air Fryer at 400 degrees F for 10 minutes, shaking the cooking basket halfway through the cooking time.
Adjust the seasonings to taste and serve immediately.

The Best Calamari Appetizer

Preparation Time: 20 minutes
Servings: 6
Nutrition: 274 Calories; 3g Fat; 38g Carbs; 29g Protein; 3g Sugars
Ingredients:
1 ½ pounds calamari tubes, cleaned, cut into rings
Sea salt and ground black pepper, to taste
2 tablespoons lemon juice
1 cup cornmeal
1 cup all-purpose flour
1 teaspoon paprika
1 egg, whisked
1/4 cup buttermilk
Directions:
Preheat your Air Fryer to 390 degrees F. Rinse the calamari and pat it dry. Season with salt and black pepper. Drizzle lemon juice all over the calamari.
Now, combine the cornmeal, flour, and paprika in a bowl; add the whisked egg and buttermilk. Dredge the calamari in the egg/flour mixture.
Arrange them in the cooking basket. Spritz with cooking oil and cook for 9 to 12 minutes, shaking the basket occasionally. Work in batches.
Serve with toothpicks. Bon appétit!

Fried Pickle Chips with Greek Yogurt Dip

Preparation Time: 20 minutes
Servings: 5
Nutrition: 138 Calories; 2g Fat; 28g Carbs; 7g Protein; 9g Sugars
Ingredients:
1/2 cup cornmeal
1/2 cup all-purpose flour
1 teaspoon cayenne pepper
1/2 teaspoon shallot powder
1 teaspoon garlic powder
1/2 teaspoon porcini powder
Kosher salt and ground black pepper, to taste
2 eggs
2 cups pickle chips, pat dry with kitchen towels
Greek Yogurt Dip:
1/2 cup Greek yogurt
1 clove garlic, minced
1/4 teaspoon ground black pepper
1 tablespoon fresh chives, chopped

Directions:
In a shallow bowl, mix the cornmeal and flour; add the seasonings and mix to combine well. Beat the eggs in a separate shallow bowl.
Dredge the pickle chips in the flour mixture, then, in the egg mixture. Press the pickle chips into the flour mixture again, coating evenly.
Cook in the preheated Air Fryer at 400 degrees F for 5 minutes; shake the basket and cook for 5 minutes more. Work in batches.
Meanwhile, mix all the sauce **Ingredients:** until well combined. Serve the fried pickles with the Greek yogurt dip and enjoy.

Teriyaki Chicken Drumettes

Preparation Time: 40 minutes
Servings: 6
Nutrition: 286 Calories; 18g Fat; 15g Carbs; 28g Protein; 11g Sugars
Ingredients:
1 ½ pounds chicken drumettes
Sea salt and cracked black pepper, to taste
2 tablespoons fresh chives, roughly chopped
Teriyaki Sauce:
1 tablespoon sesame oil
1/4 cup soy sauce
1/2 cup water
1/4 cup honey
1/2 teaspoon Five-spice powder
2 tablespoons rice wine vinegar
1/2 teaspoon fresh ginger, grated
2 cloves garlic, crushed
1 tablespoon corn starch dissolved in 3 tablespoons of water
Directions:
Start by preheating your Air Fryer to 380 degrees F. Rub the chicken drumettes with salt and cracked black pepper.
Cook in the preheated Air Fryer approximately 15 minutes. Turn them over and cook an additional 7 minutes.
While the chicken drumettes are roasting, combine the sesame oil, soy sauce, water, honey, Five-spice powder, vinegar, ginger, and garlic in a pan over medium heat. Cook for 5 minutes, stirring occasionally.
Add the cornstarch slurry, reduce the heat, and let it simmer until the glaze thickens.
After that, brush the glaze all over the chicken drumettes. Air-fry for a further 6 minutes or until the surface is crispy. Serve topped with the remaining glaze and garnished with fresh chives. Bon appétit!

Baked Cheese Crisps

Preparation Time: 15 minutes
Servings: 4
Nutrition: 198 Calories; 17g Fat; 7g Carbs; 12g Protein; 4g Sugars
Ingredients:
1/2 cup Parmesan cheese, shredded
1 cup Cheddar cheese, shredded
1 teaspoon Italian seasoning
1/2 cup marinara sauce

Directions:
Start by preheating your Air Fryer to 350 degrees F. Place a piece of parchment paper in the cooking basket.
Mix the cheese with the Italian seasoning.
Add about 1 tablespoon of the cheese mixture (per crispto the basket, making sure they are not touching. Bake for 6 minutes or until browned to your liking.
Work in batches and place them on a large tray to cool slightly. Serve with the marinara sauce. Bon appétit!

Mexican Cheesy Zucchini Bites

Preparation Time: 25 minutes
Servings: 4
Nutrition: 231 Calories; 9g Fat; 23g Carbs; 4g Protein; 3g Sugars
Ingredients:
1 large-sized zucchini, thinly sliced
1/2 cup flour
1/4 cup yellow cornmeal
1 egg, whisked
1/2 cup tortilla chips, crushed
1/2 cup Queso Añejo, grated
Salt and cracked pepper, to taste
Directions:
Pat dry the zucchini slices with a kitchen towel.
Mix the remaining **Ingredients:** in a shallow bowl; mix until everything is well combined. Dip each zucchini slice in the prepared batter.
Cook in the preheated Air Fryer at 400 degrees F for 12 minutes, shaking the basket halfway through the cooking time.
Work in batches until the zucchini slices are crispy and golden brown. Enjoy!

Bruschetta with Fresh Tomato and Basil

Preparation Time: 15 minutes
Servings: 3
Nutrition: 161 Calories; 5g Fat; 28g Carbs; 4g Protein; 5g Sugars
Ingredients:
1/2 Italian bread, sliced
2 garlic cloves, peeled
2 tablespoons extra-virgin olive oil
2 ripe tomatoes, chopped
1 teaspoon dried oregano
Salt, to taste
8 fresh basil leaves, roughly chopped
Directions:
Place the bread slices on the lightly greased Air Fryer grill pan. Bake at 370 degrees F for 3 minutes.
Cut a clove of garlic in half and rub over one side of the toast; brush with olive oil. Add the chopped tomatoes. Sprinkle with oregano and salt.
Increase the temperature to 380 degrees F. Cook in the preheated Air Fryer for 3 minutes more. Garnish with fresh basil and serve. Bon appétit!

Roasted Parsnip Sticks with Salted Caramel

Preparation Time: 25 minutes
Servings: 4
Nutrition: 213 Calories; 11g Fat; 24g Carbs; 4g Protein; 3g Sugars
Ingredients:
1 pound parsnip, trimmed, scrubbed, cut into sticks
2 tablespoon avocado oil
2 tablespoons granulated sugar
2 tablespoons butter
1/4 teaspoon ground allspice
1/2 teaspoon coarse salt
Directions:
Toss the parsnip with the avocado oil; bake in the preheated Air Fryer at 380 degrees F for 15 minutes, shaking the cooking basket occasionally to ensure even cooking.
Then, heat the sugar and 1 tablespoon of water in a small pan over medium heat. Cook until the sugar has dissolved; bring to a boil.
Keep swirling the pan around until the sugar reaches a rich caramel color. Pour in 2 tablespoons of cold water. Now, add the butter, allspice, and salt. The mixture should be runny.
Afterwards, drizzle the salted caramel over the roasted parsnip sticks and enjoy!

Greek-Style Squash Chips

Preparation Time: 25 minutes
Servings: 4
Nutrition: 180 Calories; 13g Fat; 13g Carbs; 8g Protein; 8g Sugars
Ingredients:
1/2 cup seasoned breadcrumbs
1/2 cup Parmesan cheese, grated
Sea salt and ground black pepper, to taste
1/4 teaspoon oregano
2 yellow squash, cut into slices
2 tablespoons grapeseed oil
Sauce:
1/2 cup Greek-style yogurt
1 tablespoon fresh cilantro, chopped
1 garlic clove, minced
Freshly ground black pepper, to your liking
Directions:
In a shallow bowl, thoroughly combine the seasoned breadcrumbs, Parmesan, salt, black pepper, and oregano.
Dip the yellow squash slices in the prepared batter, pressing to adhere.
Brush with the grapeseed oil and cook in the preheated Air Fryer at 400 degrees F for 12 minutes. Shake the Air Fryer basket periodically to ensure even cooking. Work in batches.
While the chips are baking, whisk the sauce **Ingredients:**; place in your refrigerator until ready to serve. Enjoy!

Romano Cheese and Broccoli Balls

Preparation Time: 25 minutes
Servings: 4
Nutrition: 192 Calories; 12g Fat; 9g Carbs; 15g Protein; 6g Sugars
Ingredients:
1/2 pound broccoli
1/2 cup Romano cheese, grated
2 garlic cloves, minced
1 shallot, chopped
4 eggs, beaten
2 tablespoons butter, at room temperature
1/2 teaspoon paprika
1/4 teaspoon dried basil
Sea salt and ground black pepper, to taste
Directions:
Add the broccoli to your food processor and pulse until the consistency resembles rice.
Stir in the remaining **Ingredients:**; mix until everything is well combined. Shape the mixture into bite-sized balls and transfer them to the lightly greased cooking basket.
Cook in the preheated Air Fryer at 375 degrees F for 16 minutes, shaking halfway through the cooking time. Serve with cocktail sticks and tomato ketchup on the side.

Summer Meatball Skewers

Preparation Time: 20 minutes
Servings: 6
Nutrition: 218 Calories; 13g Fat; 17g Carbs; 11g Protein; 5g Sugars
Ingredients:
1/2 pound ground pork
1/2 pound ground beef
1 teaspoon dried onion flakes
1 teaspoon fresh garlic, minced
1 teaspoon dried parsley flakes
Salt and black pepper, to taste
1 red pepper, 1-inch pieces
1 cup pearl onions
1/2 cup barbecue sauce
Directions:
Mix the ground meat with the onion flakes, garlic, parsley flakes, salt, and black pepper. Shape the mixture into 1-inch balls.
Thread the meatballs, pearl onions, and peppers alternately onto skewers.
Microwave the barbecue sauce for 10 seconds.
Cook in the preheated Air Fryer at 380 degrees for 5 minutes. Turn the skewers over halfway through the cooking time. Brush with the sauce and cook for a further 5 minutes. Work in batches.
Serve with the remaining barbecue sauce and enjoy!

Italian-Style Tomato-Parmesan Crisps

Preparation Time: 20 minutes
Servings: 4
Nutrition: 90 Calories; 2g Fat; 7g Carbs; 8g Protein; 1g Sugars
Ingredients:
4 Roma tomatoes, sliced
2 tablespoons olive oil
Sea salt and white pepper, to taste
1 teaspoon Italian seasoning mix
4 tablespoons Parmesan cheese, grated
Directions:
Start by preheating your Air Fryer to 350 degrees F. Generously grease the Air Fryer basket with nonstick cooking oil.
Toss the sliced tomatoes with the remaining **Ingredients:**. Transfer them to the cooking basket without overlapping.
Cook in the preheated Air Fryer for 5 minutes. Shake the cooking basket and cook an additional 5 minutes. Work in batches.
Serve with Mediterranean aioli for dipping, if desired. Bon appétit!

Southern Cheese Straws

Preparation Time: 30 minutes
Servings: 6
Nutrition: 269 Calories; 13g Fat; 16g Carbs; 4g Protein; 1g Sugars
Ingredients:
1 cup all-purpose flour
Sea salt and ground black pepper, to taste
1/4 teaspoon smoked paprika
1/2 teaspoon celery seeds
4 ounces mature Cheddar, cold, freshly grated
1 sticks butter
Directions:
Start by preheating your air Fryer to 330 degrees F. Line the Air Fryer basket with parchment paper.
In a mixing bowl, thoroughly combine the flour, salt, black pepper, paprika, and celery seeds.
Then, combine the cheese and butter in the bowl of a stand mixer. Slowly stir in the flour mixture and mix to combine well.
Then, pack the dough into a cookie press fitted with a star disk. Pipe the long ribbons of dough across the parchment paper. Then cut into six-inch lengths.
Bake in the preheated Air Fryer for 15 minutes.
Repeat with the remaining dough. Let the cheese straws cool on a rack. You can store them between sheets of parchment in an airtight container. Bon appétit!

Green Bean Crisps

Preparation Time: 20 minutes
Servings: 4
Nutrition: 164 Calories; 12g Fat; 11g Carbs; 1g Protein; 1g Sugars
Ingredients:
1 egg, beaten
1/4 cup cornmeal
1/4 cup parmesan, grated

1 teaspoon sea salt
1/2 teaspoon red pepper flakes, crushed
1 pound green beans
2 tablespoons grapeseed oil

Directions:

In a mixing bowl, combine together the egg, cornmeal, parmesan, salt, and red pepper flakes; mix to combine well.

Dip the green beans into the batter and transfer them to the cooking basket. Brush with the grapeseed oil.

Cook in the preheated Air Fryer at 390 degrees F for 4 minutes. Shake the basket and cook for a further 3 minutes. Work in batches.

Taste, adjust the seasonings and serve. Bon appétit!

Loaded Tater Tot Bites

Preparation Time: 20 minutes
Servings: 6
Nutrition: 164 Calories; 7g Fat; 2g Carbs; 3g Protein; 8g Sugars

Ingredients:

24 tater tots, frozen
1 cup Swiss cheese, grated
6 tablespoons Canadian bacon, cooked and chopped
1/4 cup Ranch dressing

Directions:

Spritz the silicone muffin cups with non-stick cooking spray. Now, press the tater tots down into each cup.

Divide the cheese, bacon, and Ranch dressing between tater tot cups.

Cook in the preheated Air Fryer at 395 degrees for 10 minutes. Serve in paper cake cups. Bon appétit!

SWEETS

Lentils Cookies

Preparation Time: 10 minutes
Cooking duration: 25 minutes
Servings: 36
Ingredients:
1 cup water
1 cup canned lentils, drained and mashed
1 cup white flour
1 teaspoon cinnamon powder
1 cup whole wheat flour
1 teaspoon baking powder
½ teaspoon nutmeg, ground
1 cup butter, soft
½ cup brown sugar
½ cup white sugar
1 egg
2 teaspoons almond extract
1 cup raisins
1 cup rolled oats
1 cup coconut, unsweetened and shredded
Direction:
In a bowl, mix white and whole wheat flour with salt, cinnamon, baking powder and nutmeg and stir.
In a bowl, mix butter with white and brown sugar and stir using your kitchen mixer for 2 minutes.
Add egg, almond extract, lentils mix, flour mix, oats, raisins and coconut and stir everything well.
Scoop tablespoons of dough on a lined baking sheet that fits your air fryer, introduce them in the fryer and cook at 350 °F for 15 minutes.
Arrange cookies on a serving platter and serve

Lentils and Dates Brownies

Preparation Time: 10 minutes
Cooking duration: 15 minutes
Servings: 8
Ingredients:
28 ounces canned lentils, rinsed and drained
12 dates
1 tablespoon honey
1 banana, peeled and chopped
½ teaspoon baking soda
4 tablespoons almond butter
2 tablespoons cocoa powder
Direction:
In your food processor, mix lentils with butter, banana, cocoa, baking soda and honey and blend really well.
Add dates, pulse a few more times, pour this into a greased pan that fits your air fryer, spread evenly, introduce in the fryer at 360 °F and bake for 15 minutes.
Take brownies mix out of the oven, cut, arrange on a platter and serve.

Maple Cupcakes

Preparation Time: 10 minutes
Cooking duration: 20 minutes
Servings: 4
Ingredients:
4 tablespoons butter
4 eggs
½ cup pure applesauce
2 teaspoons cinnamon powder
1 teaspoon vanilla extract
½ apple, cored and chopped
4 teaspoons maple syrup
¾ cup white flour
½ teaspoon baking powder
Direction:
Heat up a pan with the butter over medium heat, add applesauce, vanilla, eggs and maple syrup, stir and take off heat and leave aside to cool down.
Add flour, cinnamon, baking powder and apples, whisk, pour in a cupcake pan, introduce in your air fryer at 350 °F and bake for 20 minutes.
Leave cupcakes them to cool down, transfer to a platter and serve them.

Rhubarb Pie

Preparation Time: 30 minutes
Cooking duration: 45 minutes
Servings: 6
Ingredients:
1 and ¼ cups almond flour
8 tablespoons butter
5 tablespoons cold water
1 teaspoon sugar
For the filling:
3 cups rhubarb, chopped
3 tablespoons flour
1 and ½ cups sugar
2 eggs
½ teaspoon nutmeg, ground
1 tablespoon butter
2 tablespoons low fat milk
Direction:
In a bowl, mix 1 and ¼ cups flour with 1 teaspoon sugar, 8 tablespoons butter and cold water, stir and knead until you obtain a dough.
Transfer dough to a floured working surface, shape a disk, flatten, wrap in plastic, keep in the fridge for about 30 minutes, roll and press on the bottom of a pie pan that fits your air fryer.
In a bowl, mix rhubarb with 1 and ½ cups sugar, nutmeg, 3 tablespoons flour and whisk.
In another bowl, whisk eggs with milk, add to rhubarb mix, pour the whole mix into the pie crust, introduce in your air fryer and cook at 390 °F for 45 minutes.
Cut and serve it cold.

Lemon Tart

Preparation Time: 1 hour
Cooking duration: 35 minutes
Servings: 6
Ingredients:
For the crust:
2 tablespoons sugar
2 cups white flour
A pinch of salt
3 tablespoons ice water
12 tablespoons cold butter
For the filling:
2 eggs, whisked
1 and ¼ cup sugar
10 tablespoons melted and chilled butter
Juice from 2 lemons
Zest from 2 lemons, grated
Direction:
In a bowl, mix 2 cups flour with a pinch of salt and 2 tablespoons sugar and whisk.
Add 12 tablespoons butter and the water, knead until you obtain a dough, shape a ball, wrap in foil and keep in the fridge for 1 hour.
Transfer dough to a floured surface, flatten it, arrange on the bottom of a tart pan, prick with a fork, keep in the fridge for 20 minutes, introduce in your air fryer at 360 °F and bake for 15 minutes.
In a bowl, mix 1 and ¼ cup sugar with eggs, 10 tablespoons butter, lemon juice and lemon zest and whisk very well.
Pour this into pie crust, spread evenly, introduce in the fryer and cook at 360 °F for 20 minutes.
Cut and serve it.

Mandarin Pudding

Preparation Time: 20 minutes
Cooking duration: 40 minutes
Servings: 8
Ingredients:
1 mandarin, peeled and sliced
Juice from 2 mandarins
2 tablespoons brown sugar
4 ounces butter, soft
2 eggs, whisked
¾ cup sugar
¾ cup white flour
¾ cup almonds, ground
Honey for serving
Direction:
Grease a loaf pan with some butter, sprinkle brown sugar on the bottom and arrange mandarin slices.
In a bowl, mix butter with sugar, eggs, almonds, flour and mandarin juice, stir, spoon this over mandarin slices, place pan in your air fryer and cook at 360 °F for 40 minutes.
Transfer pudding to a plate and serve with honey on top.

Chocolate Birthday Cake

Preparation Time: 35 minutes + chilling time
Servings: 6
Nutrition: 689 Calories; 44g Fat; 71g Carbs; 5g Protein; 56g Sugars
Ingredients:
2 eggs, beaten
2/3 cup sour cream
1 cup flour
1/2 cup sugar
1/4 cup honey
1/3 cup coconut oil, softened
1/4 cup cocoa powder
2 tablespoons chocolate chips
1 ½ teaspoons baking powder
1 teaspoon vanilla extract
1/2 teaspoon pure rum extract
Chocolate Frosting:
1/2 cup butter, softened
1/4 cup cocoa powder
2 cups powdered sugar
2 tablespoons milk
Directions:
Mix all **Ingredients:** for the chocolate cake with a hand mixer on low speed. Scrape the batter into a cake pan.
Bake at 330 degrees F for 25 to 30 minutes. Transfer the cake to a wire rack
Meanwhile, whip the butter and cocoa until smooth. Stir in the powdered sugar. Slowly and gradually, pour in the milk until your frosting reaches desired consistency.
Whip until smooth and fluffy; then, frost the cooled cake. Place in your refrigerator for a couple of hours. Serve well chilled.

Favorite New York Cheesecake

Preparation Time: 40 minutes + chilling time
Servings: 8
Nutrition: 477 Calories; 32g Fat; 35g Carbs; 18g Protein; 39g Sugars
Ingredients:
1 ½ cups digestive biscuits crumbs
2 ounces white sugar
1 ounce demerara sugar
1/2 stick butter, melted
32 ounces full-fat cream cheese
1/2 cup heavy cream
1 ¼ cups caster sugar
3 eggs, at room temperature
1 tablespoon vanilla essence
1 teaspoon grated lemon zest
Directions:
Coat the sides and bottom of a baking pan with a little flour.
In a mixing bowl, combine the digestive biscuits, white sugar, and demerara sugar. Add the melted butter and mix until your mixture looks like breadcrumbs.

Press the mixture into the bottom of the prepared pan to form an even layer. Bake at 330 degrees F for 7 minutes until golden brown. Allow it to cool completely on a wire rack.
Meanwhile, in a mixer fitted with the paddle attachment, prepare the filling by mixing the soft cheese, heavy cream, and caster sugar; beat until creamy and fluffy.
Crack the eggs into the mixing bowl, one at a time; add the vanilla and lemon zest and continue to mix until fully combined.
Pour the prepared topping over the cooled crust and spread evenly.
Bake in the preheated Air Fryer at 330 degrees F for 25 to 30 minutes; leave it in the Air Fryer to keep warm for another 30 minutes.
Cover your cheesecake with plastic wrap. Place in your refrigerator and allow it to cool at least 6 hours or overnight. Serve well chilled.

English-Style Scones with Raisins

Preparation Time: 20 minutes
Servings: 6
Nutrition: 317 Calories; 19g Fat; 25g Carbs; 9g Protein; 2g Sugars
Ingredients:
1 ½ cups all-purpose flour
1/4 cup brown sugar
1 teaspoon baking powder
1/4 teaspoon sea salt
1/4 teaspoon ground cloves
1/2 teaspoon ground cardamom
1 teaspoon ground cinnamon
1/2 cup raisins
6 tablespoons butter, cooled and sliced
1/2 cup double cream
2 eggs, lightly whisked
1/2 teaspoon vanilla essence
Directions:
In a mixing bowl, thoroughly combine the flour, sugar, baking powder, salt, cloves, cardamom cinnamon, and raisins. Mix until everything is combined well.
Add the butter and mix again.
In another mixing bowl, combine the double cream with the eggs and vanilla; beat until creamy and smooth.
Stir the wet **Ingredients:** into the dry mixture. Roll your dough out into a circle and cut into wedges.
Bake in the preheated Air Fryer at 360 degrees for 11 minutes, rotating the pan halfway through the cooking time. Bon appétit!

Baked Peaches with Oatmeal Pecan Streusel

Preparation Time: 20 minutes
Servings: 3
Nutrition: 247 Calories; 11g Fat; 28g Carbs; 9g Protein; 21g Sugars
Ingredients:
2 tablespoons old-fashioned rolled oats
3 tablespoons golden caster sugar
1/2 teaspoon ground cinnamon
1 egg
2 tablespoons cold salted butter, cut into pieces
3 tablespoons pecans, chopped

3 large ripe freestone peaches, halved and pitted

Directions:

Mix the rolled oats, sugar, cinnamon, egg, and butter until well combined.

Add a big spoonful of prepared topping to the center of each peach. Pour 1/2 cup of water into an Air Fryer safe dish. Place the peaches in the dish.

Top the peaches with the roughly chopped pecans. Bake at 340 degrees F for 17 minutes. Serve at room temperature. Bon appétit!

Red Velvet Pancakes

Preparation Time: 35 minutes

Servings: 3

Nutrition: 392 Calories; 18g Fat; 50g Carbs; 8g Protein; 32g Sugars

Ingredients:

1/2 cup flour
1 teaspoon baking powder
1/4 teaspoon salt
2 tablespoons white sugar
1/2 teaspoon cinnamon
1 teaspoon red paste food color
1 egg
1/2 cup milk
1 teaspoon vanilla
Topping:
2 ounces cream cheese, softened
2 tablespoons butter, softened
3/4 cup powdered sugar

Directions:

Mix the flour, baking powder, salt, sugar, cinnamon, red paste food color in a large bowl.

Gradually add the egg and milk, whisking continuously, until well combined. Let it stand for 20 minutes.

Spritz the Air Fryer baking pan with cooking spray. Pour the batter into the pan using a measuring cup.

Cook at 230 degrees F for 4 to 5 minutes or until golden brown. Repeat with the remaining batter.

Meanwhile, make your topping by mixing the **Ingredients:** until creamy and fluffy. Decorate your pancakes with topping. Bon appétit!

Spanish-Style Doughnut Tejeringos

Preparation Time: 20 minutes

Servings: 4

Nutrition: 311 Calories; 23g Fat; 25g Carbs; 1g Protein; 4g Sugars

Ingredients:

3/4 cup water
1 tablespoon sugar
1/4 teaspoon sea salt
1/4 teaspoon grated nutmeg
1/4 teaspoon ground cloves
6 tablespoons butter
3/4 cup all-purpose flour
2 eggs

Directions:
To make the dough, boil the water in a pan over medium-high heat; now, add the sugar, salt, nutmeg, and cloves; cook until dissolved.
Add the butter and turn the heat to low. Gradually stir in the flour, whisking continuously, until the mixture forms a ball.
Remove from the heat; fold in the eggs one at a time, stirring to combine well.
Pour the mixture into a piping bag with a large star tip. Squeeze 4-inch strips of dough into the greased Air Fryer pan.
Cook at 410 degrees F for 6 minutes, working in batches. Bon appétit!

Baked Fruit Compote with Coconut Chips

Preparation Time: 25 minutes
Servings: 6
Nutrition: 215 Calories; 5g Fat; 32g Carbs; 2g Protein; 26g Sugars
Ingredients:
1 tablespoon butter
8 ounces canned apricot halves, drained
8 ounces canned pear halves, drained
16 ounces pineapple slices, undrained
1/3 cup packed brown sugar
1/4 teaspoon grated nutmeg
1/4 teaspoon ground cloves
1/2 teaspoon ground cinnamon
1 teaspoon pure vanilla extract
1/2 cup coconut chips
Directions:
Start by preheating your Air Fryer to 330 degrees F. Grease a baking pan with butter.
Place all **Ingredients:**, except for the coconut chips, in a baking pan. Bake in the preheated Air Fryer for 20 minutes.
Serve in individual bowls, garnished with coconut chips. Bon appétit!

Summer Peach Crisp

Preparation Time: 40 minutes
Servings: 4
Nutrition: 330 Calories; 16g Fat; 42g Carbs; 2g Protein; 38g Sugars
Ingredients:
2 cups fresh peaches, pitted and sliced
1/4 cup cornmeal
1/4 cup brown sugar
1 teaspoon pure vanilla extract
1/2 teaspoon ground cinnamon
A pinch of fine sea salt
1 stick cold butter
1/2 cup rolled oats
Directions:
Toss the sliced peaches with the cornmeal, brown sugar, vanilla extract, cinnamon, and sea salt. Place in a baking pan coated with cooking spray.
In a mixing dish, thoroughly combine the cold butter and rolled oats. Sprinkle the mixture over each peach.
Bake in the preheated Air Fryer at 330 degrees F for 35 minutes. Bon appétit!

Greek-Style Griddle Cakes

Preparation Time: 15 minutes
Servings: 4
Nutrition: 276 Calories; 5g Fat; 42g Carbs; 14g Protein; 14g Sugars
Ingredients:
3/4 cup self-raising flour
1/4 teaspoon fine sea salt
2 tablespoons sugar
1/2 cup milk
2 eggs, lightly beaten
1 tablespoon butter
Topping:
1 cup Greek-style yogurt
1 banana, mashed
2 tablespoons honey
Directions:
Mix the flour, salt, and sugar in a bowl. Then, stir in the milk, eggs, and butter. Mix until smooth and uniform.
Drop tablespoons of the batter into the Air Fryer pan.
Cook at 300 degrees F for 4 to 5 minutes or until bubbles form on top of the griddle cakes. Repeat with the remaining batter.
Meanwhile, mix all **Ingredients:** for the topping. Place in your refrigerator until ready to serve.
Serve the griddle cakes with the chilled topping. Enjoy!

Nana's Famous Apple Fritters

Preparation Time: 20 minutes
Servings: 4
Nutrition: 280 Calories; 7g Fat; 51g Carbs; 4g Protein; 38g Sugars
Ingredients:
2/3 cup all-purpose flour
3 tablespoons granulated sugar
A pinch of sea salt
A pinch of freshly grated nutmeg
1 teaspoon baking powder
2 eggs, whisked
1/4 cup milk
2 apples, peeled, cored and diced
1/2 cup powdered sugar
Directions:
Mix the flour, sugar, salt, nutmeg and baking powder.
In a separate bowl whisk the eggs with the milk; add this wet mixture into the dry **Ingredients:**; mix to combine well.
Add the apple pieces and mix again.
Cook in the preheated Air Fryer at 370 degrees for 3 minutes, flipping them halfway through the cooking time. Repeat with the remaining batter.
Dust with powdered sugar and serve at room temperature. Bon appétit!

Authentic Indian Gulgulas

Preparation Time: 20 minutes
Servings: 3
Nutrition: 252 Calories; 9g Fat; 48g Carbs; 9g Protein; 14g Sugars
Ingredients:
1 banana, mashed
1/4 cup sugar
1 egg
1/2 teaspoon vanilla essence
1/4 teaspoon ground cardamom
1/4 teaspoon cinnamon
1/2 milk
3/4 cup all-purpose flour
1 teaspoon baking powder
Directions:
In a mixing bowl, whisk the mashed banana with the sugar and egg; add the vanilla, cardamom, and cinnamon and mix to combine well.
Gradually pour in the milk and mix again. Stir in the flour and baking powder. Mix until everything is well incorporated.
Drop a spoonful of batter onto the greased Air Fryer pan. Cook in the preheated Air Fryer at 360 degrees F for 5 minutes, flipping them halfway through the cooking time.
Repeat with the remaining batter and serve warm. Enjoy!

Coconut Pancake Cups

Preparation Time: 30 minutes
Servings: 4
Nutrition: 274 Calories; 13g Fat; 26g Carbs; 7g Protein; 5g Sugars
Ingredients:
1/2 cup flour
1/3 cup coconut milk
2 eggs
1 tablespoon coconut oil, melted
1 teaspoon vanilla
A pinch of ground cardamom
1/2 cup coconut chips
Directions:
Mix the flour, coconut milk, eggs, coconut oil, vanilla, and cardamom in a large bowl.
Let it stand for 20 minutes. Spoon the batter into a greased muffin tin.
Cook at 230 degrees F for 4 to 5 minutes or until golden brown. Repeat with the remaining batter.
Decorate your pancakes with coconut chips. Bon appétit!

Salted Caramel Cheesecake

Preparation Time: 1 hour + chilling time
Servings: 10
Nutrition: 501 Calories; 33g Fat; 36g Carbs; 1g Protein; 22g Sugars
Ingredients:
1 cup granulated sugar
1/3 cup water
3/4 cup heavy cream
2 tablespoons butter

1 teaspoon vanilla extract
1/2 teaspoon coarse sea salt
Crust:
1 ½ cups graham cracker crumbs
1/3 cup salted butter, melted
2 tablespoons brown sugar
Topping:
20 ounces cream cheese, softened
1 cup sour cream
1 cup granulated sugar
1 teaspoon vanilla essence
1/4 teaspoon ground star anise
3 eggs

Directions:

To make the caramel sauce, cook the sugar in a saucepan over medium heat; shake it to form a flat layer.

Add the water and cook until the sugar dissolves. Raise the heat to medium-high, and continue to cook your caramel for a further 10 minutes until it turns amber colored.

Turn the heat off; immediately stir in the heavy cream, butter, vanilla extract, and salt. Stir to combine well.

Let the salted caramel sauce cool to room temperature.

Beat all **Ingredients:** for the crust in a mixing bowl. Press the mixture into the bottom of a lightly greased baking pan.

Bake at 350 degrees F for 18 minutes. Place it in your freezer for 20 minutes.

Then, make the cheesecake topping by mixing the remaining **Ingredients:**. Pour the prepared topping over the cooled crust and spread evenly.

Bake in the preheated Air Fryer at 330 degrees F for 25 to 30 minutes; leave it in the Air Fryer to keep warm for another 30 minutes.

Refrigerate your cheesecake until completely cool and firm or overnight. Prior to serving, pour the salted caramel sauce over the cheesecake. Bon appétit!

Banana Crepes with Apple Topping

Preparation Time: 40 minutes
Servings: 2
Nutrition: 367 Calories; 11g Fat; 57g Carbs; 12g Protein; 46g Sugars
Ingredients:
Banana Crepes:
1 large banana, mashed
2 eggs, beaten
1/4 teaspoon baking powder
1 shot dark rum
1/2 teaspoon vanilla extract
1 teaspoon butter, melted
2 tablespoons brown sugar
Topping:
2 apples, peeled, cored, and chopped
2 tablespoons sugar
1/2 teaspoon cinnamon
3 tablespoons water

Directions:

Mix all **Ingredients:** for the banana crepes until creamy and fluffy. Let it stand for 15 to 20 minutes.

Spritz the Air Fryer baking pan with cooking spray. Pour the batter into the pan using a measuring cup.

Cook at 230 degrees F for 4 to 5 minutes or until golden brown. Repeat with the remaining batter.

To make the pancake topping, place all **Ingredients:** in a heavy-bottomed skillet over medium heat. Cook for 10 minutes, stirring occasionally. Spoon on top of the banana crepes and enjoy!

Apricot and Walnut Crumble

Preparation Time: 40 minutes
Servings: 8
Nutrition: 404 Calories; 14g Fat; 62g Carbs; 6g Protein; 51g Sugars
Ingredients:

2 pounds apricots, pitted and sliced
1 cup brown sugar
2 tablespoons cornstarch
Topping:
1 ½ cups old-fashioned rolled oats
½ cup brown sugar
2 tablespoons agave nectar
1 teaspoon crystallized ginger
½ teaspoon ground cardamom
A pinch of salt
1 stick butter, cut into pieces
1/2 cup walnuts, chopped
1/2 cup dried cranberries

Directions:

Toss the sliced apricots with the brown sugar and cornstarch. Place in a baking pan lightly greased with nonstick cooking spray.

In a mixing dish, thoroughly combine all the topping **Ingredients:**. Sprinkle the topping **Ingredients:** over the apricot layer.

Bake in the preheated Air Fryer at 330 degrees F for 35 minutes. Bon appétit!

Butter Rum Cookies with Walnuts

Preparation Time: 35 minutes
Servings: 6
Nutrition: 364 Calories; 29g Fat; 23g Carbs; 9g Protein; 7g Sugars
Ingredients:

1 cup all-purpose flour
1/2 teaspoon baking powder
1/4 teaspoon fine sea salt
1 stick butter, unsalted and softened
1/2 cup sugar
1 egg
1/2 teaspoon vanilla
1 teaspoon butter rum flavoring
3 ounces walnuts, finely chopped

Directions:

Begin by preheating the Air Fryer to 360 degrees F.

In a mixing dish, thoroughly combine the flour with baking powder and salt.

Beat the butter and sugar with a hand mixer until pale and fluffy; add the whisked egg, vanilla, and butter rum flavoring; mix again to combine well. Now, stir in the dry **Ingredients:**.
Fold in the chopped walnuts and mix to combine. Divide the mixture into small balls; flatten each ball with a fork and transfer them to a foil-lined baking pan.
Bake in the preheated Air Fryer for 14 minutes. Work in a few batches and transfer to wire racks to cool completely. Bon appétit!

Classic Butter Cake

Preparation Time: 35 minutes
Servings: 8
Nutrition: 244 Calories; 12g Fat; 21g Carbs; 2g Protein; 18g Sugars
Ingredients:
1 stick butter, at room temperature
1 cup sugar
2 eggs
1 cup all-purpose flour
1 teaspoon baking powder
1/2 teaspoon baking soda
1/4 teaspoon salt
A pinch of freshly grated nutmeg
A pinch of ground star anise
1/4 cup buttermilk
1 teaspoon vanilla essence
Directions:
Begin by preheating your Air Fryer to 320 degrees F. Spritz the bottom and sides of a baking pan with cooking spray.
Beat the butter and sugar with a hand mixer until creamy. Then, fold in the eggs, one at a time, and mix well until fluffy.
Stir in the flour along with the remaining **Ingredients:**. Mix to combine well. Scrape the batter into the prepared baking pan.
Bake for 15 minutes; rotate the pan and bake an additional 15 minutes, until the top of the cake springs back when gently pressed with your fingers. Bon appétit!

Pecan Fudge Brownies

Preparation Time: 30 minutes
Servings: 6
Nutrition: 341 Calories; 25g Fat; 33g Carbs; 2g Protein; 12g Sugars
Ingredients:
1/2 cup butter, melted
1/2 cup sugar
1 teaspoon vanilla essence
1 egg
1/2 cup flour
1/2 teaspoon baking powder
1/4 cup cocoa powder
1/2 teaspoon ground cinnamon
1/4 teaspoon fine sea salt
1 ounce semisweet chocolate, coarsely chopped
1/4 cup pecans, finely chopped
Directions:
Start by preheating your Air Fryer to 350 degrees F. Now, lightly grease six silicone molds.

In a mixing dish, beat the melted butter with the sugar until fluffy. Next, stir in the vanilla and egg and beat again.
After that, add the flour, baking powder, cocoa powder, cinnamon, and salt. Mix until everything is well combined.
Fold in the chocolate and pecans; mix to combine. Bake in the preheated Air Fryer for 20 to 22 minutes. Enjoy!

Fried Honey Banana

Preparation Time: 20 minutes
Servings: 2
Nutrition: 363 Calories; 13g Fat; 61g Carbs; 7g Protein; 33g Sugars
Ingredients:
2 ripe bananas, peeled and sliced
2 tablespoons honey
3 tablespoons rice flour
3 tablespoons desiccated coconut
A pinch of fine sea salt
1/2 teaspoon baking powder
1/4 teaspoon cardamom powder
Directions:
Preheat the Air Fryer to 390 degrees F.
Drizzle honey over the banana slices.
In a mixing dish, thoroughly combine the rice flour, coconut, salt, baking powder, and cardamom powder. Roll each slice of banana over the flour mixture.
Bake in the preheated Air Fryer approximately 13 minutes, flipping them halfway through the cooking time. Bon appétit!

Pop Tarts with Homemade Strawberry Jam

Preparation Time: 45 minutes
Servings: 8
Nutrition: 173 Calories; 9g Fat; 21g Carbs; 6g Protein; 7g Sugars
Ingredients:
1 cup strawberries, sliced
1 tablespoon fresh lemon juice
1 teaspoon maple syrup
2 tablespoons chia seeds
1 (14-ouncebox refrigerated pie crust
1 egg, whisked with 1 tablespoon of water (egg wash
1/2 cup powdered sugar
Directions:
In a saucepan, heat the strawberries until they start to get syrupy. Mash them and add the lemon juice and maple syrup.
Remove from the heat and stir in the chia seeds. Let it stand for 30 minutes or until it thickens up.
Unroll the pie crusts and cut them into small rectangles. Spoon the strawberry jam in the center of a rectangle; top with another piece of crust.
Repeat until you run out of **Ingredients:**. Line the Air Fryer basket with parchment paper.
Brush the pop tarts with the egg wash and bake at 400 degrees F for 6 minutes or until slightly brown. Work in batches and transfer to cooling racks.
Dust with powdered sugar and enjoy!

Fall Harvest Apple Cinnamon Buns

Preparation Time: 1 hour 20 minutes
Servings: 6
Nutrition: 430 Calories; 13g Fat; 61g Carbs; 8g Protein; 25g Sugars
Ingredients:
1/2 cup milk
1/2 cup granulated sugar
1 tablespoon yeast
1/2 stick butter, at room temperature
1 egg, at room temperature
1/4 teaspoon salt
2 ¼ cups all-purpose flour
Filling:
3 tablespoons butter, at room temperature
1/4 cup brown sugar
1/2 teaspoon ground cardamom
1/2 teaspoon ground cloves
1 teaspoon ground cinnamon
1 apple, peeled, cored, and chopped
1/2 cup powdered sugar
Directions:
Heat the milk in a microwave safe bowl and transfer the warm milk to the bowl of a stand electric mixer. Add the granulated sugar and yeast, and mix to combine well. Cover and let sit until the yeast is foamy.
Then, beat the butter on low speed. Fold in the the egg and mix again. Add the salt and flour. Mix on medium speed until a soft dough forms.
Knead the dough on a lightly floured surface. Cover it loosely and let sit in a warm place about 1 hour or until doubled in size. Then, spritz the bottom and sides of a baking pan with cooking oil (butter flavored).
Roll your dough out into a rectangle.
Spread 3 tablespoons of butter all over the dough. In a mixing dish, combine the brown sugar, cardamom, cloves, and cinnamon; sprinkle evenly over the dough.
Top with the chopped apples. Then, roll up your dough to form a log. Cut into 6 equal rolls and place them in the parchment-lined Air Fryer basket.
Bake at 350 degrees for 12 minutes, turning them halfway through the cooking time. Dust with powdered sugar. Bon appétit!

Pear Fritters with Cinnamon and Ginger

Preparation Time: 20 minutes
Servings: 4
Nutrition: 333 Calories; 5g Fat; 52g Carbs; 15g Protein; 19g Sugars
Ingredients:
2 pears, peeled, cored and sliced
1 tablespoon coconut oil, melted
1 ½ cups all-purpose flour
1 teaspoon baking powder
A pinch of fine sea salt
A pinch of freshly grated nutmeg
1/2 teaspoon ginger
1 teaspoon cinnamon

2 eggs
4 tablespoons milk
Directions:
Mix all **Ingredients:**, except for the pears, in a shallow bowl. Dip each slice of the pears in the batter until well coated.
Cook in the preheated Air Fryer at 360 degrees for 4 minutes, flipping them halfway through the cooking time. Repeat with the remaining **Ingredients:**.
Dust with powdered sugar if desired. Bon appétit!

Old-Fashioned Plum Dumplings

Preparation Time: 40 minutes
Servings: 4
Nutrition: 395 Calories; 12g Fat; 55g Carbs; 1g Protein; 37g Sugars
Ingredients:
1 (14-ouncebox pie crusts
2 cups plums, pitted
2 tablespoons granulated sugar
2 tablespoons coconut oil
1/4 teaspoon ground cardamom
1/2 teaspoon ground cinnamon
1 egg white, slightly beaten
Directions:
Place the pie crust on a work surface. Roll into a circle and cut into quarters.
Place 1 plum on each crust piece. Add the sugar, coconut oil, cardamom, and cinnamon. Roll up the sides into a circular shape around the plums.
Repeat with the remaining **Ingredients:**. Brush the edges with the egg white. Place in the lightly greased Air Fryer basket.
Bake in the preheated Air Fryer at 360 degrees F for 20 minutes, flipping them halfway through the cooking time. Work in two batches, decorate and serve at room temperature. Bon appétit!

Almond Chocolate Cupcakes

Preparation Time: 20 minutes
Servings: 6
Nutrition: 288 Calories; 17g Fat; 31g Carbs; 1g Protein; 20g Sugars
Ingredients:
3/4 cup self-raising flour
1 cup powdered sugar
1/4 teaspoon salt
1/4 teaspoon nutmeg, preferably freshly grated
1 tablespoon cocoa powder
2 ounces butter, softened
1 egg, whisked
2 tablespoons almond milk
1/2 teaspoon vanilla extract
1 ½ ounces dark chocolate chunks
1/2 cup almonds, chopped
Directions:
In a mixing bowl, combine the flour, sugar, salt, nutmeg, and cocoa powder. Mix to combine well.
In another mixing bowl, whisk the butter, egg, almond milk, and vanilla.

Now, add the wet egg mixture to the dry **Ingredients:**. Then, carefully fold in the chocolate chunks and almonds; gently stir to combine.
Scrape the batter mixture into muffin cups. Bake your cupcakes at 350 degrees F for 12 minutes until a toothpick comes out clean.
Decorate with chocolate sprinkles if desired. Serve and enjoy!

Almond Cupcakes

Preparation Time: 5 minutes
Cooking time: 25 minutes
Servings: 4
Ingredients:
1/3 cup coconut flour
½ cup cocoa powder
3 tablespoons stevia
½ teaspoon baking soda
1 teaspoon baking powder
4 eggs, whisked
1 teaspoon vanilla extract
4 tablespoons coconut oil, melted
¼ cup almond milk
Cooking spray
Directions:
In a bowl, mix all the **Ingredients:** except the cooking spray and whisk well.
Grease a cupcake tin that fits the air fryer with the cooking spray, pour the cupcake mix, put the pan in your air fryer, cook at 350 degrees F for 25 minutes, cool down and serve.
Nutrition: calories 103, fat 4, fiber 2, carbs 6, protein 3

Coconut Cookies

Preparation Time: 5 minutes
Cooking time: 15 minutes
Servings: 8
Ingredients:
1 and ½ cups coconut, shredded
2 tablespoons erythritol
½ teaspoon baking powder
¼ teaspoon almond extract
2 eggs, whisked
Directions:
In a bowl, mix all the **Ingredients:** and whisk well.
Scoop 8 servings of this mix on a baking sheet that fits the air fryer which you've lined with parchment paper.
Put the baking sheet in your air fryer and cook at 350 degrees F for 15 minutes.
Serve cold.
Nutrition: calories 125, fat 7, fiber 1, carbs 5, protein 4

Coconut Bars

Preparation Time: 5 minutes
Cooking time: 40 minutes
Servings: 12
Ingredients:
1 and ¼ cups almond flour

1 cup swerve
1 cup butter, melted
½ cup coconut cream
1 and ½ cups coconut, flaked
1 egg yolk
¾ cup walnuts, chopped
½ teaspoon vanilla extract

Directions:

In a bowl, mix the flour with half of the swerve and half of the butter, stir well and press this on the bottom of a baking pan that fits the air fryer.

Introduce this in the air fryer and cook at 350 degrees F for 15 minutes.

Meanwhile, heat up a pan with the rest of the butter over medium heat, add the remaining swerve and the rest of the **Ingredients:**, whisk, cook for 1-2 minutes, take off the heat and cool down.

Spread this well over the crust, put the pan in the air fryer again and cook at 350 degrees F for 25 minutes.

Cool down, cut into bars and serve.

Nutrition: calories 182, fat 12, fiber 2, carbs 4, protein 4

Lemon Bars

Preparation Time: 10 minutes
Cooking time: 35 minutes
Servings: 8
Ingredients:

½ cup butter, melted
1 cup erythritol
1 and ¾ cups almond flour
3 eggs, whisked
Zest of 1 lemon, grated
Juice of 3 lemons

Directions:

In a bowl, mix 1 cup flour with half of the erythritol and the butter, stir well and press into a baking dish that fits the air fryer lined with parchment paper.

Put the dish in your air fryer and cook at 350 degrees F for 10 minutes.

Meanwhile, in a bowl, mix the rest of the flour with the remaining erythritol and the other **Ingredients:** and whisk well.

Spread this over the crust, put the dish in the air fryer once more and cook at 350 degrees F for 25 minutes.

Cool down, cut into bars and serve.

Nutrition: calories 210, fat 12, fiber 1, carbs 4, protein 8

Sweet Zucchini Bread

Preparation Time: 10 minutes
Cooking time: 40 minutes
Servings: 12
Ingredients:

2 cups almond flour
2 teaspoons baking powder
¾ cup swerve
½ cup coconut oil, melted
1 teaspoon lemon juice
1 teaspoon vanilla extract

3 eggs, whisked
1 cup zucchini, shredded
1 tablespoon lemon zest
Cooking spray

Directions:

In a bowl, mix all the **Ingredients:** except the cooking spray and stir well.

Grease a loaf pan that fits the air fryer with the cooking spray, line with parchment paper and pour the loaf mix inside.

Put the pan in the air fryer and cook at 330 degrees F for 40 minutes.

Cool down, slice and serve.

Nutrition: calories 143, fat 11, fiber 1, carbs 3, protein 3

Lemon Coconut Pie

Preparation Time: 10 minutes
Cooking time: 35 minutes
Servings: 8

Ingredients:

2 eggs, whisked
¾ cup swerve
¼ cup coconut flour
2 tablespoons butter, melted
1 teaspoon lemon zest, grated
1 teaspoon baking powder
1 teaspoon vanilla extract
½ teaspoon lemon extract
4 ounces coconut, shredded
Cooking spray

Directions:

In a bowl, combine all the **Ingredients:** except the cooking spray and stir well.

Grease a pie pan that fits the air fryer with the cooking spray, pour the mixture inside, put the pan in the air fryer and cook at 360 degrees F for 35 minutes.

Slice and serve warm.

Nutrition: calories 212, fat 15, fiber 2, carbs 6, protein 4

Strawberry Tart

Preparation Time: 5 minutes
Cooking time: 20 minutes
Servings: 8

Ingredients:

5 egg whites
1/3 cup swerve
1 and ½ cups almond flour
Zest of 1 lemon, grated
1 teaspoon baking powder
1 teaspoon vanilla extract
1/3 cup butter, melted
2 cups strawberries, sliced
Cooking spray

Directions:

In a bowl, whisk egg whites well.

Add the rest of the **Ingredients:** except the cooking spray gradually and whisk everything.

Grease a tart pan with the cooking spray, and pour the strawberries mix.
Put the pan in the air fryer and cook at 370 degrees F for 20 minutes.
Cool down, slice and serve.
Nutrition: calories 182, fat 12, fiber 1, carbs 6, protein 5

Coconut Donuts

Preparation Time: 5 minutes
Cooking time: 15 minutes
Servings: 4
Ingredients:
8 ounces coconut flour
2 tablespoons stevia
1 egg, whisked
2 and ½ tablespoons butter, melted
4 ounces coconut milk
1 teaspoon baking powder
Directions:
In a bowl, mix all the **Ingredients:** and whisk well.
Shape donuts from this mix, place them in your air fryer's basket and cook at 370 degrees F for 15 minutes.
Serve warm.
Nutrition: calories 190, fat 12, fiber 1, carbs 4, protein 6

Butter Cookies

Preparation Time: 10 minutes
Cooking time: 20 minutes
Servings: 12
Ingredients:
2 eggs, whisked
1 tablespoon heavy cream
½ cup butter, melted
2 teaspoons vanilla extract
2 and ¾ cup almond flour
Cooking spray
¼ cup swerve
Directions:
In a bowl, mix all the **Ingredients:** except the cooking spray and stir well.
Shape 12 balls out of this mix, put them on a baking sheet that fits the air fryer greased with cooking spray and flatten them.
Put the baking sheet in the air fryer and cook at 350 degrees F for 20 minutes.
Serve the cookies cold.
Nutrition: calories 234, fat 13, fiber 2, carbs 4, protein 7

Ginger Cookies

Preparation Time: 10 minutes
Cooking time: 15 minutes
Servings: 12
Ingredients:
2 cups almond flour
1 cup swerve
¼ cup butter, melted

1 egg
2 teaspoons ginger, grated
1 teaspoon vanilla extract
¼ teaspoon nutmeg, ground
¼ teaspoon cinnamon powder

Directions:

In a bowl, mix all the **Ingredients:** and whisk well.

Spoon small balls out of this mix on a lined baking sheet that fits the air fryer lined with parchment paper and flatten them.

Put the sheet in the fryer and cook at 360 degrees F for 15 minutes.

Cool the cookies down and serve.

Nutrition: calories 220, fat 13, fiber 2, carbs 4, protein 3

Raspberry Muffins

Preparation Time: 10 minutes
Cooking time: 20 minutes
Servings: 8
Ingredients:

¾ cup raspberries
¼ cup ghee, melted
1 egg
½ cup swerve
¼ cup coconut flour
2 tablespoons almond meal
1 teaspoon cinnamon powder
3 tablespoons cream cheese
½ teaspoon baking soda
½ teaspoon baking powder
Cooking spray

Directions:

In a bowl, mix all the **Ingredients:** except the cooking spray and whisk well.

Grease a muffin pan that fits the air fryer with the cooking spray, pour the raspberry mix, put the pan in the machine and cook at 350 degrees F for 20 minutes.

Serve the muffins cold.

Nutrition: calories 223, fat 7, fiber 2, carbs 4, protein 5

Strawberry Jam

Preparation Time: 10 minutes
Cooking time: 20 minutes
Servings: 12
Ingredients:

¼ cup swerve
8 ounces strawberries, sliced
1 tablespoon lemon juice
¼ cup water

Directions:

In a pan that fits the air fryer, combine all the **Ingredients:**, put the pan in the machine and cook at 380 degrees F for 20 minutes.

Divide the mix into cups, cool down and serve.

Nutrition: calories 100, fat 1, fiber 0, carbs 1, protein 1

Blueberry Cream

Preparation Time: 4 minutes
Cooking time: 20 minutes
Servings: 6
Ingredients:
2 cups blueberries
Juice of ½ lemon
2 tablespoons water
1 teaspoon vanilla extract
2 tablespoons swerve
Directions:
In a bowl, mix all the **Ingredients:** and whisk well.
Divide this into 6 ramekins, put them in the air fryer and cook at 340 degrees F for 20 minutes
Cool down and serve.
Nutrition: calories 123, fat 2, fiber 2, carbs 4, protein 3

Cocoa Cake

Preparation Time: 5 minutes
Cooking time: 20 minutes
Servings: 8
Ingredients:
2 egg
3 tablespoons swervef
3 tablespoons coconut oil, melted
¼ cup coconut milk
4 tablespoons almond flour
1 tablespoon cocoa powder
½ teaspoon baking powder
Directions:
In a bowl, mix all the **Ingredients:** and stir well.
Pour this into a cake pan that fits the air fryer, put the pan in the machine and cook at 340 degrees F for 20 minutes.
Slice and serve.
Nutrition: calories 191, fat 12, fiber 2, carbs 4, protein 6

Blackberry Chia Jam

Preparation Time: 10 minutes
Cooking time: 30 minutes
Servings: 12
Ingredients:
3 cups blackberries
¼ cup swerve
4 tablespoons lemon juice
4 tablespoons chia seeds
Directions:
In a pan that fits the air fryer, combine all the **Ingredients:** and toss.
Put the pan in the machine and cook at 300 degrees F for 30 minutes.
Divide into cups and serve cold.
Nutrition: calories 100, fat 2, fiber 1, carbs 3, protein 1

Mixed Berries Cream

Preparation Time: 5 minutes
Cooking time: 30 minutes
Servings: 6
Ingredients:
12 ounces blackberries
6 ounces raspberries
12 ounces blueberries
¾ cup swerve
2 ounces coconut cream
Directions:
In a bowl, mix all the **Ingredients:** and whisk well.
Divide this into 6 ramekins, put them in your air fryer and cook at 320 degrees F for 30 minutes.
Cool down and serve it.
Nutrition: calories 100, fat 1, fiber 1, carbs 2, protein 2

Cream Cheese Brownies

Preparation Time: 10 minutes
Cooking time: 25 minutes
Servings: 6
Ingredients:
6 tablespoons cream cheese, soft
3 eggs, whisked
2 tablespoons cocoa powder
3 tablespoons coconut oil, melted
¼ cup almond flour
¼ cup coconut flour
¼ teaspoon baking soda
1 teaspoon vanilla extract
½ cup almond milk
3 tablespoons swerve
Cooking spray
Directions:
Grease a cake pan that fits the air fryer with the cooking spray.
In a bowl, mix rest of the **Ingredients:**, whisk well and pour into the pan.
Put the pan in your air fryer, cook at 370 degrees F for 25 minutes, cool the brownies down, slice and serve.
Nutrition: calories 182, fat 12, fiber 2, carbs 4, protein 6

Tasty Banana Cake

Preparation Time: 10 minutes
Cooking duration: 30 minutes
Servings: 4
Ingredients:
1 tablespoon butter, soft
1 egg
1/3 cup brown sugar
2 tablespoons honey
1 banana, peeled and mashed
1 cup white flour

1 teaspoon baking powder
½ teaspoon cinnamon powder
Cooking spray
Direction:
Spray a cake pan with some cooking spray and leave aside.
In a bowl, mix butter with sugar, banana, honey, egg, cinnamon, baking powder and flour and whisk
Pour this into a cake pan greased with cooking spray, introduce in your air fryer and cook at 350 °F for 30 minutes.
Leave cake to cool down, slice and serve.

Simple Cheesecake

Preparation Time: 10 minutes
Cooking duration: 15 minutes
Servings: 15
Ingredients:
1 pound cream cheese
½ teaspoon vanilla extract
2 eggs
4 tablespoons sugar
1 cup graham crackers, crumbled
2 tablespoons butter
Direction:
In a bowl, mix crackers with butter.
Press crackers mix on the bottom of a lined cake pan, introduce in your air fryer and cook at 350 °F for 4 minutes.
Meanwhile, in a bowl, mix sugar with cream cheese, eggs and vanilla and whisk well.
Spread filling over crackers crust and cook your cheesecake in your air fryer at 310 °F for 15 minutes.
Leave cake in the fridge for 3 hours, slice and serve.

Bread Pudding

Preparation Time: 10 minutes
Cooking duration: 1 hour
Servings: 4
Ingredients:
6 glazed doughnuts, crumbled
1 cup cherries
4 egg yolks
1 and ½ cups whipping cream
½ cup raisins
¼ cup sugar
½ cup chocolate chips.
Direction:
In a bowl, mix cherries with egg yolks and whipping cream and stir well.
In another bowl, mix raisins with sugar, chocolate chips and doughnuts and stir.
Combine the 2 mixtures, transfer everything to a greased pan that fits your air fryer and cook at 310 °F for 1 hour.
Chill pudding before cutting and serving it.

Bread Dough and Amaretto Dessert

Preparation Time: 10 minutes
Cooking duration: 12 minutes
Servings: 12
Ingredients:
1 pound bread dough
1 cup sugar
½ cup butter, melted
1 cup heavy cream
12 ounces chocolate chips
2 tablespoons amaretto liqueur
Direction:
Roll dough, cut into 20 slices and then cut each slice in halves.
Brush dough pieces with butter, sprinkle sugar, place them in your air fryer's basket after you've brushed it some butter, cook them at 350 °F for 5 minutes, flip them, cook for 3 minutes more and transfer to a platter.
Heat up a pan with the heavy cream over medium heat, add chocolate chips and stir until they melt.
Add liqueur, stir again, transfer to a bowl and serve bread dippers with this sauce.

Cinnamon Rolls and Cream Cheese Dip

Preparation Time: 2 hours
Cooking duration: 15 minutes
Servings: 8
Ingredients:
1 pound bread dough
¾ cup brown sugar
1 and ½ tablespoons cinnamon, ground
¼ cup butter, melted
For the cream cheese dip:
2 tablespoons butter
4 ounces cream cheese
1 and ¼ cups sugar
½ teaspoon vanilla
Direction:
Roll dough on a floured working surface, shape a rectangle and brush with ¼ cup butter.
In a bowl, mix cinnamon with sugar, stir, sprinkle this over dough, roll dough into a log, seal well and cut into 8 pieces.
Leave rolls to rise for 2 hours, place them in your air fryer's basket, cook at 350 °F for 5 minutes, flip them, cook for 4 minutes more and transfer to a platter.
In a bowl, mix cream cheese with butter, sugar and vanilla and whisk really well.
Serve your cinnamon rolls with this cream cheese dip.

Pumpkin Pie

Preparation Time: 10 minutes
Cooking duration: 15 minutes
Servings: 9
Ingredients:
1 tablespoon sugar
2 tablespoons flour

1 tablespoon butter
2 tablespoons water
For the pumpkin pie filling:5 ounces pumpkin flesh, chopped
1 teaspoon mixed spice
1 teaspoon nutmeg
3 ounces water
1 egg, whisked
1 tablespoon sugar
Direction:
Put 3 ounces water in a pot, bring to a boil over medium high heat, add pumpkin, egg, 1 tablespoon sugar, spice and nutmeg, stir, boil for 20 minutes, take off heat and blend using an immersion blender.
In a bowl, mix flour with butter, 1 tablespoon sugar and 2 tablespoons water and knead your dough well.
Grease a pie pan that fits your air fryer with butter, press dough into the pan, fill with pumpkin pie filling, place in your air fryer's basket and cook at 360 °F for 15 minutes.
Slice and serve warm.

Wrapped Pears

Preparation Time: 10 minutes
Cooking duration: 15 minutes
Servings: 4
Ingredients:
4 puff pastry sheets
14 ounces vanilla custard
2 pears, halved
1 egg, whisked
½ teaspoon cinnamon powder
2 tablespoons sugar
Direction:
Place puff pastry slices on a working surface, add spoonful of vanilla custard in the center of each, top with pear halves and wrap.
Brush pears with egg, sprinkle sugar and cinnamon, place them in your air fryer's basket and cook at 320 °F for 15 minutes.
Divide parcels on plates and serve.

Strawberry Donuts

Preparation Time: 10 minutes
Cooking duration: 15 minutes
Servings: 4
Ingredients:
8 ounces flour
1 tablespoon brown sugar
1 tablespoon white sugar
1 egg
2 and ½ tablespoons butter
4 ounces whole milk
1 teaspoon baking powder
For the strawberry icing:
2 tablespoons butter
5 ounces icing sugar

½ teaspoon pink coloring
¼ cup strawberries, chopped
1 tablespoon whipped cream
Direction:
In a bowl, mix butter, 1 tablespoon brown sugar, 1 tablespoon white sugar and flour and stir.
In a second bowl, mix egg with 1 and ½ tablespoons butter and milk and stir well.
Combine the 2 mixtures, stir, shape donuts from this mix, and place them in your air fryer's basket and cook at 360 °F for 15 minutes.
Put 1 tablespoon butter, icing sugar, food coloring, whipped cream and strawberry puree and whisk well.
Arrange donuts on a platter and serve with strawberry icing on top.

Air Fried Bananas

Preparation Time: 10 minutes
Cooking duration: 15 minutes
Servings: 4
Ingredients:
3 tablespoons butter
2 eggs
8 bananas, peeled and halved
½ cup corn flour
3 tablespoons cinnamon sugar
1 cup panko
Direction:
Heat up a pan with the butter over medium high heat, add panko, stir and cook for 4 minutes and then transfer to a bowl.
Roll each in flour, eggs and panko mix, arrange them in your air fryer's basket, dust with cinnamon sugar and cook at 280 °F for 10 minutes.
Serve right away.

Cocoa Cake

Preparation Time: 10 minutes
Cooking duration: 17 minutes
Servings: 6
Ingredients:
5 ounces butter, melted
3 eggs
3 ounces sugar
1 teaspoon cocoa powder
3 ounces flour
½ teaspoon lemon juice
Direction:
In a bowl, mix 1 tablespoon butter with cocoa powder and whisk.
In another bowl, mix the rest of the butter with sugar, eggs, flour and lemon juice, whisk well and pour half into a cake pan that fits your air fryer.
Add half of the cocoa mix, spread, add the rest of the butter layer and top with the rest of cocoa.
Introduce in your air fryer and cook at 360 °F for 17 minutes.
Cool cake down before slicing and serving.

Chocolate Cake

Preparation Time: 10 minutes
Cooking duration: 30 minutes
Servings: 12
Ingredients:

¾ cup white flour
¾ cup whole wheat flour
1 teaspoon baking soda
¾ teaspoon pumpkin pie spice
¾ cup sugar
1 banana, mashed
½ teaspoon baking powder
2 tablespoons canola oil
½ cup Greek yogurt
8 ounces canned pumpkin puree
Cooking spray
1 egg
½ teaspoon vanilla extract
2/3 cup chocolate chips

Direction:

In a bowl, mix white flour with whole wheat flour, salt, baking soda and powder and pumpkin spice and stir.
In another bowl, mix sugar with oil, banana, yogurt, pumpkin puree, vanilla and egg and stir using a mixer.
Combine the 2 mixtures, add chocolate chips, stir, pour this into a greased Bundt pan that fits your air fryer.
Introduce in your air fryer and cook at 330 °F for 30 minutes.
Leave the cake to cool down, before cutting and serving it.

Apple Bread

Preparation Time: 10 minutes
Cooking duration: 40 minutes
Servings: 6
Ingredients:

3 cups apples, cored and cubed
1 cup sugar
1 tablespoon vanilla
2 eggs
1 tablespoon apple pie spice
2 cups white flour
1 tablespoon baking powder
1 stick butter
1 cup water

Direction:

In a bowl mix egg with 1 butter stick, apple pie spice and sugar and stir using your mixer.
Add apples and stir again well.
In another bowl, mix baking powder with flour and stir.
Combine the 2 mixtures, stir and pour into a spring form pan.
Put spring form pan in your air fryer and cook at 320 °F for 40 minutes
Slice and serve.

Banana Bread

Preparation Time: 10 minutes
Cooking duration: 40 minutes
Servings: 6
Ingredients:
¾ cup sugar
1/3 cup butter
1 teaspoon vanilla extract
1 egg
2 bananas, mashed
1 teaspoon baking powder
1 and ½ cups flour
½ teaspoons baking soda
1/3 cup milk
1 and ½ teaspoons cream of tartar
Cooking spray
Direction:
In a bowl, mix milk with cream of tartar, sugar, butter, egg, vanilla and bananas and stir everything.
In another bowl, mix flour with baking powder and baking soda.
Combine the 2 mixtures, stir well, pour this into a cake pan greased with some cooking spray, introduce in your air fryer and cook at 320 °F for 40 minutes.
Take bread out, leave aside to cool down, slice and serve it.

Mini Lava Cakes

Preparation Time: 10 minutes
Cooking duration: 20 minutes
Servings: 3
Ingredients:
1 egg
4 tablespoons sugar
2 tablespoons olive oil
4 tablespoons milk
4 tablespoons flour
1 tablespoon cocoa powder
½ teaspoon baking powder
½ teaspoon orange zest
Direction:
In a bowl, mix egg with sugar, oil, milk, flour, salt, cocoa powder, baking powder and orange zest, stir very well and pour this into greased ramekins.
Add ramekins to your air fryer and cook at 320 °F for 20 minutes.
Serve lava cakes warm.

Crispy Apple

Preparation Time: 10 minutes
Cooking duration: 10 minutes
Servings: 4
Ingredients:
2 teaspoons cinnamon powder
5 apples, cored and cut into chunks

½ teaspoon nutmeg powder
1 tablespoon maple syrup
½ cup water
4 tablespoons butter
¼ cup flour
¾ cup old fashioned rolled oats
¼ cup brown sugar

Direction:

Put the apples in a pan that fits your air fryer, add cinnamon, nutmeg, maple syrup and water.
In a bowl, mix butter with oats, sugar, salt and flour, stir, drop spoonful of this mix on top of apples, introduce in your air fryer and cook at 350 °F for 10 minutes.
Serve warm.

Carrot Cake

Preparation Time: 10 minutes
Cooking duration: 45 minutes
Servings: 6
Ingredients:

5 ounces flour
¾ teaspoon baking powder
½ teaspoon baking soda
½ teaspoon cinnamon powder
¼ teaspoon nutmeg, ground
½ teaspoon allspice
1 egg
3 tablespoons yogurt
½ cup sugar
¼ cup pineapple juice
4 tablespoons sunflower oil
1/3 cup carrots, grated
1/3 cup pecans, toasted and chopped
1/3 cup coconut flakes, shredded
Cooking spray

Direction:

In a bowl, mix flour with baking soda and powder, salt, allspice, cinnamon and nutmeg and stir.
In another bowl, mix egg with yogurt, sugar, pineapple juice, oil, carrots, pecans and coconut flakes and stir well.
Combine the two mixtures and stir well, pour this into a spring form pan that fits your air fryer which you've greased with some cooking spray, transfer to your air fryer and cook on 320 °F for 45 minutes.
Leave cake to cool down, then cut and serve it.

Ginger Cheesecake

Preparation Time: 2 hours and 10 minutes
Cooking duration: 20 minutes
Servings: 6
Ingredients:

2 teaspoons butter, melted
½ cup ginger cookies, crumbled
16 ounces cream cheese, soft
2 eggs

½ cup sugar
1 teaspoon rum
½ teaspoon vanilla extract
½ teaspoon nutmeg, ground

Direction:

Grease a pan with the butter and spread cookie crumbs on the bottom.

In a bowl, beat cream cheese with nutmeg, vanilla, rum and eggs, whisk well and spread over the cookie crumbs.

Introduce in your air fryer and cook at 340 °F for 20 minutes.

Leave cheesecake to cool down and keep in the fridge for 2 hours before slicing and serving it.

Strawberry Pie

Preparation Time: 10 minutes
Cooking duration: 20 minutes
Servings: 12
Ingredients:

For the crust:
1 cup coconut, shredded
1 cup sunflower seeds
¼ cup butter

For the filling:
1 teaspoon gelatin
8 ounces cream cheese
4 ounces strawberries
2 tablespoons water
½ tablespoon lemon juice
¼ teaspoon stevia
½ cup heavy cream
8 ounces strawberries, chopped for serving

Direction:

In your food processor, mix sunflower seeds with coconut, a pinch of salt and butter, pulse and press this on the bottom of a cake pan that fits your air fryer.

Heat up a pan with the water over medium heat, add gelatin, stir until it dissolves, leave aside to cool down, add this to your food processor, mix with 4 ounces strawberries, cream cheese, lemon juice and stevia and blend well.

Add heavy cream, stir well and spread this over crust.

Top with 8 ounces strawberries, introduce in your air fryer and cook at 330 °F for 15 minutes.

Keep in the fridge until you serve it.

Coffee Cheesecakes

Preparation Time: 10 minutes
Cooking duration: 20 minutes
Servings: 6
Ingredients:

For the cheesecakes:
2 tablespoons butter
8 ounces cream cheese
3 tablespoons coffee
3 eggs
1/3 cup sugar
1 tablespoon caramel syrup

For the frosting:
3 tablespoons caramel syrup
3 tablespoons butter
8 ounces mascarpone cheese, soft
2 tablespoons sugar
Direction:
In your blender, mix cream cheese with eggs, 2 tablespoons butter, coffee, 1 tablespoon caramel syrup and 1/3 cup sugar and pulse very well, spoon into a cupcakes pan that fits your air fryer, introduce in the fryer and cook at 320 °F and bake for 20 minutes.
Leave aside to cool down and then keep in the freezer for 3 hours.
Meanwhile, in a bowl, mix 3 tablespoons butter with 3 tablespoons caramel syrup, 2 tablespoons sugar and mascarpone, blend well, spoon this over cheesecakes and serve them.

Cocoa Cookies

Preparation Time: 10 minutes
Cooking duration: 14 minutes
Servings: 12
Ingredients:
6 ounces coconut oil, melted
6 eggs
3 ounces cocoa powder
2 teaspoons vanilla
½ teaspoon baking powder
4 ounces cream cheese
5 tablespoons sugar
Direction:
In a blender, mix eggs with coconut oil, cocoa powder, baking powder, vanilla, cream cheese and swerve and stir using a mixer.
Pour this into a lined baking dish that fits your air fryer, introduce in the fryer at 320 °F and bake for 14 minutes.
Slice cookie sheet into rectangles and serve.

Special Brownies

Preparation Time: 10 minutes
Cooking duration: 17 minutes
Servings: 4
Ingredients:
1 egg
1/3 cup cocoa powder
1/3 cup sugar
7 tablespoons butter
½ teaspoon vanilla extract
¼ cup white flour
¼ cup walnuts, chopped
½ teaspoon baking powder
1 tablespoon peanut butter
Direction:
Heat up a pan with 6 tablespoons butter and the sugar over medium heat, stir, cook for 5 minutes, transfer this to a bowl, add salt, vanilla extract, cocoa powder, egg, baking powder, walnuts and flour, stir the whole thing really well and pour into a pan that fits your air fryer.

In a bowl, mix 1 tablespoon butter with peanut butter, heat up in your microwave for a few seconds, stir well and drizzle this over brownies mix.
Introduce in your air fryer and bake at 320 °F and bake for 17 minutes.
Leave brownies to cool down, cut and serve.

Blueberry Scones

Preparation Time: 10 minutes
Cooking duration: 10 minutes
Servings: 10
Ingredients:
1 cup white flour
1 cup blueberries
2 eggs
½ cup heavy cream
½ cup butter
5 tablespoons sugar
2 teaspoons vanilla extract
2 teaspoons baking powder
Direction:
In a bowl, mix flour, salt, baking powder and blueberries and stir.
In another bowl, mix heavy cream with butter, vanilla extract, sugar and eggs and stir well.
Combine the 2 mixtures, knead until you obtain your dough, shape 10 triangles from this mix, place them on a lined baking sheet that fits your air fryer and cook them at 320 °F for 10 minutes.
Serve them cold.

Chocolate Cookies

Preparation Time: 10 minutes
Cooking duration: 25 minutes
Servings: 12
Ingredients:
1 teaspoon vanilla extract
½ cup butter
1 egg
4 tablespoons sugar
2 cups flour
½ cup unsweetened chocolate chips
Direction:
Heat up a pan with the butter over medium heat, stir and cook for 1 minute.
In a bowl, mix egg with vanilla extract and sugar and stir well.
Add melted butter, flour and half of the chocolate chips and stir everything.
Transfer this to a pan that fits your air fryer, spread the rest of the chocolate chips on top, introduce in the fryer at 330 °F and bake for 25 minutes.
Slice when it's cold and serve.

Tasty Orange Cake

Preparation Time: 10 minutes
Cooking duration: 32 minutes
Servings: 12
Ingredients:
6 eggs
1 orange, peeled and cut into quarters

1 teaspoon vanilla extract
1 teaspoon baking powder
9 ounces flour
2 ounces sugar+ 2 tablespoons
2 tablespoons orange zest
4 ounces cream cheese
4 ounces yogurt

Direction:

In your food processor, pulse orange very well.

Add flour, 2 tablespoons sugar, eggs, baking powder, vanilla extract and pulse well again.

Transfer this into 2 spring form pans, introduce each in your fryer and cook at 330 °F for 16 minutes.

Meanwhile, in a bowl, mix cream cheese with orange zest, yogurt and the rest of the sugar and stir well.

Place one cake layer on a plate, add half of the cream cheese mix, add the other cake layer and top with the rest of the cream cheese mix.

Spread it well, slice and serve.

Macaroons

Preparation Time: 10 minutes
Cooking duration: 8 minutes
Servings: 20
Ingredients:
2 tablespoons sugar
4 egg whites
2 cup coconut, shredded
1 teaspoon vanilla extract

Direction:

In a bowl, mix egg whites with stevia and beat using your mixer.

Add coconut and vanilla extract, whisk again, shape small balls out of this mix, introduce them in your air fryer and cook at 340 °F for 8 minutes.

Serve macaroons cold.

Lime Cheesecake

Preparation Time: 4 hours and 10 minutes
Cooking duration: 4 minutes
Servings: 10
Ingredients:
2 tablespoons butter, melted
2 teaspoons sugar
4 ounces flour
¼ cup coconut, shredded

For the filling:
1 pound cream cheese
Zest from 1 lime, grated
Juice form 1 lime
2 cups hot water
2 sachets lime jelly

Direction:

In a bowl, mix coconut with flour, butter and sugar, stir well and press this on the bottom of a pan that fits your air fryer.

Meanwhile, put the hot water in a bowl, add jelly sachets and stir until it dissolves.
Put cream cheese in a bowl, add jelly, lime juice and zest and whisk really well.
Add this over the crust, spread, introduce in the air fryer and cook at 300 °F for 4 minutes.
Keep in the fridge for 4 hours before serving.

Easy Granola

Preparation Time: 10 minutes
Cooking duration: 35 minutes
Servings: 4
Ingredients:
1 cup coconut, shredded
½ cup almonds
½ cup pecans, chopped
2 tablespoons sugar
½ cup pumpkin seeds
½ cup sunflower seeds
2 tablespoons sunflower oil
1 teaspoon nutmeg, ground
1 teaspoon apple pie spice mix
Direction:
In a bowl, mix almonds and pecans with pumpkin seeds, sunflower seeds, coconut, nutmeg and apple pie spice mix and stir well.
Heat up a pan with the oil over medium heat, add sugar and stir well.
Pour this over nuts and coconut mix and stir well.
Spread this on a lined baking sheet that fits your air fryer, introduce in your air fryer and cook at 300 °F and bake for 25 minutes.
Leave your granola to cool down, cut and serve.

Strawberry Cobbler

Preparation Time: 10 minutes
Cooking duration: 25 minutes
Servings: 6
Ingredients:
¾ cup sugar
6 cups strawberries, halved
1/8 teaspoon baking powder
1 tablespoon lemon juice
½ cup flour
A pinch of baking soda
½ cup water
3 and ½ tablespoon olive oil
Cooking spray
Direction:
In a bowl, mix strawberries with half of sugar, sprinkle some flour, add lemon juice, whisk and pour into the baking dish that fits your air fryer and greased with cooking spray
In another bowl, mix flour with the rest of the sugar, baking powder and soda and stir well.
Add the olive oil and mix until the whole thing with your hands.
Add ½ cup water and spread over strawberries.
Introduce in the fryer at 355 °F and bake for 25 minutes.
Leave cobbler aside to cool down, slice and serve.

Black Tea Cake

Preparation Time: 10 minutes
Cooking duration: 35 minutes
Servings: 12
Ingredients:
6 tablespoons black tea powder
2 cups milk
½ cup butter
2 cups sugar
4 eggs
2 teaspoons vanilla extract
½ cup olive oil
3 and ½ cups flour
1 teaspoon baking soda
3 teaspoons baking powder
For the cream:
6 tablespoons honey
4 cups sugar
1 cup butter, soft
Direction:
Put the milk in a pot, heat up over medium heat, add tea, stir well, take off heat and leave aside to cool down.
In a bowl, mix ½ cup butter with 2 cups sugar, eggs, vegetable oil, vanilla extract, baking powder, baking soda and 3 and ½ cups flour and stir everything really well.
Pour this into 2 greased round pans, introduce each in the fryer at 330 °F and bake for 25 minutes.
In a bowl, mix 1 cup butter with honey and 4 cups sugar and stir really well.
Arrange one cake on a platter, spread the cream all over, top with the other cake and keep in the fridge until you serve it.

Plum Cake

Preparation Time: 1 hour and 20 minutes
Cooking duration: 36 minutes
Servings: 8
Ingredients:
7 ounces flour
1 package dried yeast
1 ounce butter, soft
1 egg, whisked
5 tablespoons sugar
3 ounces warm milk
1 and ¾ pounds plums, pitted and cut into quarters Zest from 1 lemon, grated
1 ounce almond flakes
Direction:
In a bowl, mix yeast with butter, flour and 3 tablespoons sugar and stir well.
Add milk and egg and whisk for 4 minutes until your obtain a dough.
Arrange the dough in a spring form pan that fits your air fryer and which you've greased with some butter, cover and leave aside for 1 hour.
Arrange plumps on top of the butter, sprinkle the rest of the sugar, introduce in your air fryer at 350 °F, bake for 36 minutes, cool down, sprinkle almond flakes and lemon zest on top, slice and serve.

CPSIA information can be obtained
at www.ICGtesting.com
Printed in the USA
LVHW050343180121
676772LV00011B/370

9 781914 253324